Clinical Methods in Study of Cholesterol Metabolism

Monographs on Atherosclerosis

Vol. 9

Editors
David Kritchevsky, Philadelphia, Pa.
O.J. Pollak, Dover, Del.

S. Karger · Basel · München · Paris · London · New York · Sydney

Clinical Methods in Study of Cholesterol Metabolism

H.S. Sodhi, Davis and Sacramento, Calif.
B.J. Kudchodkar, Davis, Calif.
D.T. Mason, Davis and Sacramento, Calif.

17 figures and 2 tables, 1979

S. Karger · Basel · München · Paris · London · New York · Sydney

Monographs on Atherosclerosis

Vol. 6: *William T. Beher* (Detroit, Mich.): Bile Acids. Chemistry and Physiology of Bile Acids and their Influence on Atherosclerosis. XIV + 226 p., 11 fig., 9 tab., 1976.
ISBN 3-8055-2242-8

Vol. 7: *G.A. Gresham* (Cambridge): Primate Atherosclerosis. VIII + 102 p., 6 fig., 1976.
ISBN 3-8055-2270-3

Vol. 8: *H. Engelberg* (Beverly Hills, Calif.): Heparin
R.W. Robinson; I.N. Likar, and *L.J. Likar* (Worcester, Mass.): Arterial Mast Cells
VIII + 116 p., 2 fig., 6 tab., 1978.
ISBN 3-8055-2892-2

National Library of Medicine Cataloging in Publication
Sodhi, H. S.
Clinical methods in study of cholesterol metabolism
H. S. Sodhi, B. J. Kudchodkar, D. T. Mason. – Basel, New York, Karger, 1979.
(Monographs on atherosclerosis; v. 9)
1. Cholesterol – metabolism I. Kudchodkar, B. J. II. Mason, Dean T., 1932–
III. Title IV. Series
W1 M0569T v. 9/QU 95 S679c
ISBN 3-8055-2986-4

© Copyright 1979 by S. Karger AG, 4011 Basel (Switzerland), Arnold-Böcklin-Strasse 25
Printed in Switzerland by Buchdruckerei G. Krebs AG, Basel
ISBN 3-8055-2986-4

Contents

Contents

Acknowledgments

The idea for this monograph was suggested by Dr. *D. Kritchevsky* and we are thankful for his interest and encouragement during its completion.

This manuscript represents the outcome of the work of many investigators; notably that of Drs. *E.H. Ahrens, Jr., S.M. Grundy, T. Miettinen* and *D.S. Goodman*. They developed the most reliable methods for studies on cholesterol metabolism in man which have since become the gold standards for comparing other methods.

Most of what is given in this book is based on the experience in our own research laboratories. Our thanks are due to the following former and present colleagues: Drs. *L. Horlick, G.S. Sundaram, D.J. Nazir, P.V. Varnghese, A. Salel, C. Clifford* and *Y. Terai*.

Technical and editorial assistance of Miss *Leslie Silvernail*, Mrs. *Bonnie Fulton* and Miss *Raya Drahun* is gratefully acknowledged.

Our research was supported inpart by grants from the Medical Research Council of Canada; Canadian and Saskatchewan Heart Foundations; the Ayerst Laboratories; Mead Johnson, Canada Ltd.; Research Program Project Grant HL 4780 from the National Heart, Lung and Blood Institute, NIH, Bethesda, Md.

Dedicated to the Memory of *R. Gordon Gould*, PhD
A Lifelong Student of Cholesterol Metabolism

Introduction

Cholesterol is one of the structural components of all cellular and intra-cellular membranes in the human body. Of the 140 g or so of cholesterol present in the entire body, less than 7% is present in the plasma [90, 286], and clinically this small fraction of the total body cholesterol is perhaps the most important. Patients with high levels of plasma cholesterol tend to have a much greater risk of heart attacks as compared to those with relatively lower levels of plasma cholesterol [232], and evidence accumulated in recent studies suggests that reduction of plasma cholesterol may reduce the risk of death from myocardial infarction [6, 289]. Although there is general agreement that it would be better to lower plasma levels of cholesterol, there is no unanimity of opinion as to the best way to achieve this objective.

It is generally believed that increased levels of plasma cholesterol are associated with increased rates of deposition of cholesterol in tissues including the site of atherosclerotic lesion: the arterial intima. Smoking and hypertension are other factors which influence the rate of progress of atherosclerotic changes [119, 233]. Attempts to decrease plasma cholesterol by diet or drugs are based on the hope that reduction in the rates of deposition of cholesterol may decrease both the size of the lesions as well as the risk of myocardial infarction. The observations that the cholesterol deposits in the tendons and subcutaneous tissues reduce in size when plasma cholesterol concentrations are decreased tend to support this hope. However, the relationships, if any, between the atherosclerotic lesions and the deposits of cholesterol in tendons or other body pools are not known. There is no information whether the rates of deposition in the atherosclerotic lesions or its removal from those lesions parallel the changes in the cholesterol pools in tendons or other body tissues. It is not even known that any observed reduction in mortality and morbidity from complications of atherosclerosis is mediated through an actual reduction in the cholesterol deposits in atherosclerotic lesions.

Despite extensive studies on cholesterol metabolism over the last few decades, a large number of questions still remain unanswered. The methods for reliable studies in man have become available only recently and they have remained difficult and time-consuming. Extensive data from animal studies cannot be indiscriminately extrapolated to man. There is a pressing need for more work in man and simpler methods are badly needed to facilitate this.

The primary objective of this book is to introduce various methods currently available for the study of cholesterol metabolism in man. The theoretical as well as practical aspects of these methods are given in adequate details for those interested in the study of cholesterol metabolism. No attempt has been made to deal extensively with all aspects which bear directly or indirectly on the chemistry of these methods. However, there should be no difficulty in the understanding and the execution of these methods if details (and sometimes references) given here are followed.

It is recognized that knowledge of metabolism of plasma lipoproteins (and of the methods involved) is also necessary for a proper perspective on cholesterol metabolism. Adequate recent reviews on this subject are available and therefore it has not been dealt with in this small volume. It is, however, recommended that the student of cholesterol metabolism should be thoroughly familiar with the metabolism (and structure) of plasma lipoproteins.

Chapter I. Chemistry of Cholesterol

Historical Background

Cholesterol was discovered as the major component of gallstones in the 18th century, and *De Fourcroy* [107] was among the first to prepare large quantities of a crystalline substance from extracts of human gallstones in the latter half of the century. *Chevreul* [83, 84] showed that the substance remained unchanged after boiling with potassium hydroxide, and he coined the word 'cholesterine' (from Greek 'cole', bile; 'steros', solid). This substance was then identified in human and animal bile and also in the human brain. It was later identified in hen's eggs and gradually was recognized as a normal constituent of all animal cells. In 1859, 'cholesterine' was identified as an alcohol by *Berthelot* [34] and he prepared esters of it. Later, in 1896, *Hürthle* [220] isolated cholesterol esters CE) from serum, and in 1910 *Windaus* [504] showed that the cholesterol in the atheromatous lesions was present chiefly as esters.

The credit for the elucidation of the structure of cholesterol goes mainly to *Windaus* and his associates [503–506]. In 1919, he proposed a tentative formula for cholesterol which was subsequently changed in 1932 to the one now accepted (fig. 1).

Related Steroids

The term 'steroid' is applied to compounds containing perhydrocyclopentaophenanthrene carbon skeleton. The four closed carbon rings are identified as A, B, C, and D, and the numbering of carbon atoms in the molecule is continued from the rings to the side chain (fig. 1). Cholesterol has a hydroxyl group (OH) at carbon position 3 and a double bond between carbons 5 and 6 [41, 140].

Although cholesterol is the most abundant steroid in the mammalian tissues, small quantities of other compounds related in structure to choles-

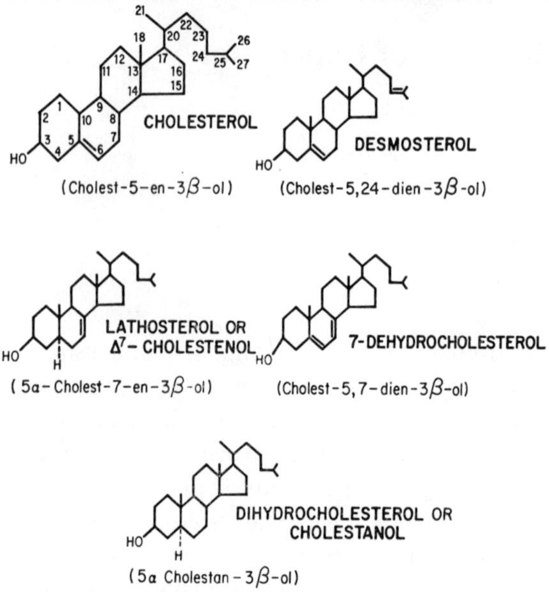

Fig. 1. Structure of cholesterol and some of the related steroids present in animal tissues.

terol are also present. A precursor of vitamin D, 7-dehydrocholesterol, has a structure almost identical to that of cholesterol in that it has only one additional double bond at carbons 7 and 8 (fig. 1), and it can be converted to vitamin D by ultraviolet (UV) irradiation of skin [35, 52].

Dihydrocholesterol or cholestanol which differs from cholesterol and lathosterol in that it has no double bond in its ring structure and $\Delta 7$-cholestenol or lathosterol (which has a double bond between carbons 7 and 8) (fig. 1) are also present in trace quantities [136–138, 298]. The bile acids, cholic and chenodeoxycholic acid, are the two primary bile acids derived from cholesterol [31, 44]. Cholesterol is also converted to a large number of steroidal hormones, such as progesterone, androgens, estrogens, adrenal cortical hormones, etc. [42, 196, 516].

Comparable steroidal compounds present in plants are generically known as 'phytosterols'. Campesterol (C28), stigmasterol (C29), and β-sitosterol (C29) are the most abundant of the plant sterols (fig. 2). Since these sterols can be absorbed, albeit only to a small extent [170, 390], they are also found in trace amounts in human tissues.

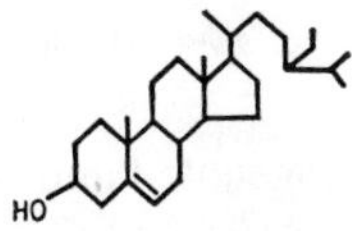

β- SITOSTEROL
(Cholest- 5-en-24-ethyl-β-ol)

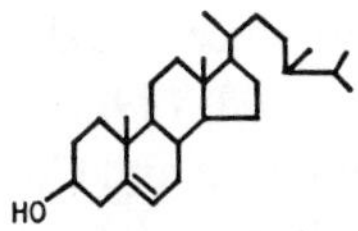

CAMPESTEROL
(Cholest-5-en-24-methyl-3β-ol)

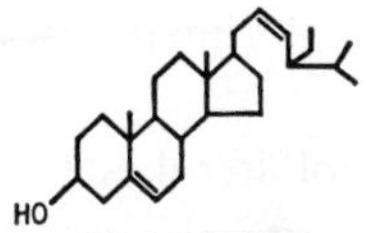

STIGMASTEROL
(Cholest-5,22-dien-24-ethyl-3β-ol)

Fig. 2. Structure of the major plant sterols present in human diet.

Physical and Chemical Properties of Cholesterol

Both the ring structure and the aliphatic side chain of cholesterol are nonpolar. The 3-β-hydroxyl group is the only polar group in the cholesterol molecule. It is, therefore, relatively insoluble in water and quite soluble in organic solvents. Its solubility in ethanol is much less than in diethyl ether [41]. Cholesterol is solid at room temperature. Its melting point is 149.5–150°C [137, 138]. It can be distilled under high vacuum and can also be sublimed. Since there are several asymmetric carbon atoms, solutions of cholesterol exhibit optical rotation which can aid in the identification and in ascertaining the purity of cholesterol preparations [41]. When crystallized from anhydrous organic solvents, it forms triclinic needles, and when crystallized from 95% alcoholic solution it separates as monohydrate, rhomb-shaped triclinic plates, which lose water at 70–80°C [41].

A variable fraction of cholesterol is present in the human body as CE [220, 347]. The fatty acids forming CE are long chain fatty acids generally containing 16–20 carbon atoms. A smaller quantity of shorter or longer chain fatty acids may also form CE in the body. The esterification of cholesterol with fatty acids occurs at the 3β position. Since the only polar group present in the free cholesterol is lost on the formation of esters, CE are essentially nonpolar.

The glycoside digitonin, the saponins tigonin and gitonin, and the alkaloid tomatine, interact with the 3β-hydroxyl group of cholesterol and precipitate with cholesterol. The reaction is specific for sterols containing the 3β-hydroxyl group, and since CE do not have the 3β-hydroxyl group, they cannot be precipitated [108, 149, 503].

The double bond between C5 and C6 can be hydrogenated and halogenated. The formation of halide, especially dibromide, has been of great practical use in purifying cholesterol obtained from natural sources [138]. Interaction between cholesterol and sulphuric acid yields intensely colored compounds and this has been the basis of a number of colorimetric assays [73, 262, 391].

Cholesterol occurs either as free alcohol or as cholesterol esterified with one of the many long chain fatty acids. In a sense, cholesterol is never present in the body as 'free' cholesterol since it is always present as a component of macromolecular complexes called lipoproteins. The 'free' cholesterol implies that it is not esterified. The bulk (approximately 80–90%) of cholesterol present in most tissues is free sterol [90]. Red blood cells (RBC) and the nervous system contain little if any of CE, while cholesterol in plasma and adrenals is present predominantly as esters [4, 50].

Other sterols, such as 7-dehydrocholesterol, dihydrocholesterol (cholestanol), etc., are present in tissues in small but variable quantities. Their concentrations in plasma are negligible; thus, their contamination does not significantly affect the quantitation of cholesterol in plasma. However, in some experiments involving the determination of specific activity (SA) of cholesterol after administration of radioactive precursors, it may be necessary to remove these (radioactive) contaminants and purify cholesterol.

Chapter II. Isolation, Purification, and Estimation of Cholesterol

The most common source of samples containing cholesterol in clinical practice is plasma or serum. For experimental studies also, the plasma and its various lipoprotein fractions are the most important sources of information. However, in some experiments, it may be necessary to analyze diet, feces, bile, and tissues for their cholesterol content.

Collection, Handling, and Storage of Samples

Collection of Blood

The concentration of plasma cholesterol is not markedly altered during the absorptive phase, but the triglycerides are significantly increased after a fatty meal. For that reason, the subjects are advised not to take anything but water for 14–16 h before the collection of blood samples. It is necessary to stop the medication known to affect the lipid metabolism for a few weeks before taking the blood samples. Other drugs taken by the subject should also be noted.

Plasma volume and concentrations of certain blood constituents change with the change in posture. When a subject stands upright from a recumbent position the plasma volume decreases, and the reverse happens when the subject changes from an upright to a recumbent position. The change in plasma volume has been attributed to the outward movement of fluid due to an increase in hydrostatic pressure [135, 490, 515]. *Stoker et al.* [451] reported that 15 min after healthy subjects changed from a recumbent to an upright position, the plasma cholesterol concentration increased by 12.5%. These findings have been confirmed by *Tan et al.* [470] who also showed that the concentration of plasma triglycerides increased by 12.4% when subjects changed from a lying to a standing position. Subjects assuming a sitting instead of an upright position showed similar but smaller changes in the concentrations of plasma lipids. Since the magnitude of these changes is similar to those observed after treatment with some hypolipidemic agents, these studies indicate the necessity of standardizing the postural position for collection of blood. Ideally, blood samples should be collected 15 min after the subject has maintained a sitting position. In any case, posture should be constant for a given subject during a given study, and one should wait at least a fixed interval of a few minutes in that posture before blood is collected.

Application of a tourniquet for 5 min or longer can also cause comparable increases in the concentration of plasma cholesterol [235, 342], although its application for less than a minute does not significantly affect plasma lipids [470]. In collecting blood samples, the tourniquet should be released immediately after the needle is placed inside the vein and the blood samples should be withdrawn after a few seconds.

Blood samples should be drawn from an antecubital vein or from some other convenient arm vein. Vacutainer tubes containing solid EDTA are convenient for collection of 1–25 ml of blood. The instructions for collections are generally supplied with the system. Use of solid EDTA as an anticoagulant eliminates dilution which could occur with tubes containing solutions of EDTA in saline. EDTA not only serves as an anticoagulant but also has the additional advantage of chelating divalent metallic ions that promote the autooxidation of lipids [366]. Other anticoagulants, such as heparin, could also be used [185, 198]. However, the blood should be kept below 10 °C and the processing of the sample should not be unduly delayed.

Samples can also be drawn directly in syringes wetted with an anticoagulant. Immediately after sampling, the blood should be transferred to tubes containing an anticoagulant. Prior to the transfer of blood into test tubes, the needles must be removed to prevent hemolysis. Once filled, the contents of the tubes must be mixed promptly by inverting 7–8 times. Mixing must be thorough but not vigorous. Blood is then placed in a refrigerator (4 °C) or in an ice bath pending separation of plasma [103, 320].

Normal blood contains an enzyme (lecithin: cholesterol acyltransferase or LCAT) which esterifies plasma free cholesterol (FC) [153]. Thus, the ratios of plasma FC to esterified cholesterol may change significantly during storage of plasma at room temperature. If blood samples contain radioactive cholesterol then the SA of plasma CE may also change as a result of the activity of this enzyme. The SA of FC may change due to exchange of FC between RBC and plasma lipoproteins [187]. Both the activity of the enzyme and exchange of FC between plasma and RBC decrease to insignificant levels at low temperatures [434]. Therefore, it is necessary not only to keep the samples at or about 4 °C, but that the plasma should be separated from cells in a refrigerated centrifuge as soon as possible after collection of the

blood. The activity of LCAT could be inhibited by adding reagents such as
p-hydroxymercuribenzoate, iodoacetate, N-ethyl maleimide, etc. [153], or by
keeping the samples chilled. The latter also reduces the risk of autooxidation
of plasma lipids.

Separation of Plasma
The tubes containing blood are centrifuged at 4 °C in a refrigerated
centrifuge for 15–20 min at 1,600 g [192, 319]. Plasma is promptly removed
from the sedimented cells using a Pasteur pipette with a rubber bulb, taking
care that plasma is not drawn in the bulb. It is transferred into a screw cap
tube and stored in the dark at 4 °C after adding inhibitors of LCAT enzyme,
if necessary.

For more details on collection and handling of blood, the reader is
referred to the *Manual of Laboratory Operations for Lipid and Lipoprotein
Analysis* [266].

Separation of Plasma Lipoproteins
Except in rare instances (type I and type V hyperlipoproteinemia), fasting samples of plasma do not contain chylomicra. If chylomicra are present,
they will float to the top when stored overnight in a refrigerator. Alternatively, they can be removed by centrifugation at 26,000 g for 30 min or 100,000 g
for 10 min [264].

The isolation of different plasma lipoproteins can be carried out by a
number of procedures. The most commonly used techniques for isolating
major lipoprotein classes is preparative ultracentrifugation and is described
briefly below. For more details, the reader is referred to several excellent
reviews [132, 194, 264].

Preparative Ultracentrifugation of Plasma Lipoproteins
The procedure as developed by *Lindgren* and his associates [263, 264] is
described below and is based on the use of the Beckman Preparative Ultra-
centrifuge, Model L2–65.

The plasma samples used for separation of the lipoproteins should
either be fresh or stored at 4 °C for less than 5 days. The samples must not
be frozen. If stored at 4 °C, plasma samples should be equilibrated at room
temperature for at least 45 min before centrifugation.

Preparative ultracentrifugation involves raising the density of 'the background' solutions of lipoproteins either by adding solid salt or by mixing
salt solutions of known density. The most commonly used salts are NaCl

for isolating low density and a mixture of NaCl and NaBr for isolating high density lipoproteins. All salt solutions should contain EDTA 100 mg/l.

The lipoproteins are classified according to the density of the background solution from which they are floated. Very low density lipoproteins (VLDL) are floated at d <1.006 g/ml, intermediate density lipoproteins (IDL) at d = 1.006–1.019 g/ml, low density lipoproteins (LDL) at d = 1.019–1.063 g/ml, and high density lipoproteins (HDL) at d = 1.063–1.21 g/ml.

Generally, the VLDL, LDL, and HDL are removed sequentially from the same plasma sample. Chylomicra (Svedberg flotation [Sf] >400) are rarely present in fasting samples, and if necessary they can be removed in a preliminary step by centrifuging at 100,000 g for 10 min at 23 °C in a 60 ti rotor or by centrifuging in a Beckman SW41 ti rotor at 1.6×10^6 g/min. VLDL are separated as follows. 4 ml plasma is transferred into a 6-ml cellulose nitrate tube and overlayered with exact amount of 0.196 m NaCl to yield a final volume of 6 ml. After centrifugation at 40,000 rpm for 18 h at 18 °C, VLDL are quantitatively removed in the upper 1-ml fraction. The second 1-ml fraction is taken to check the background density. The 4-ml bottom fraction is mixed thoroughly with a glass stirring rod and the contents quantitatively transferred to a new preparative tube. 2 ml of salt solution (0.196 M NaCl, 0.5052 M NaBr, d = 1.0435 g/ml, $N_D26 = 1.3405$) is then added and the total volume is adjusted to exactly 6 ml. This yields a salt background density (before centrifugation) of d = 1.019 g/ml. After centrifugation as above, IDL are quantitatively obtained in the top of the 1-ml fraction and another 1 ml is taken as background. The bottom 4-ml fraction is mixed thoroughly and the contents quantitatively transferred to a new preparative tube. 2 ml of the salt solution (0.196 M NaCl, 2.433 M NaBr, d = 1.1816 g/ml, $N_D26 = 1.3644$) is then added, and the total volume is adjusted to exactly 6 ml using the same salt solution. The centrifugal conditions are the same as above. After the run is complete, LDL (d = 1.063 g/ml) are quantitatively obtained in the top of 1 ml fraction and another 1 ml is taken as a background. The bottom 4 ml is then throroughly mixed again and transferred to a new preparative cellulose nitrate tube. 2 ml of 0.196 M NaCl, 7.572 M NaBr (d = 1.4744 g/ml, $N_D = 1.4120$) is added and mixed. This yields a salt background (before centrifugation) of d = 1.216 g/ml. Centrifuge at 40,000 rpm for 24–26 h. The total HDL are removed in the top of 1 ml fraction and 0.5 ml of the fraction is taken as reference background.

When removing the samples from centrifuge, great care should be exercised to avoid any abrupt movement of the rotor or of the tubes. A special thin-walled Pasteur pipette with an inside bore of 0.4–0.6 mm should be used (Microchemical Specialties, Berkeley, Calif.). To allow visualization of the lipoproteins by their Tyndall scattering, pipetting should be done in a darkroom on a fixture equipped with a focusing light beam [265].

Isolation of Plasma Lipoproteins by Precipitation Method

All major classes of plasma lipoproteins may be precipitated at neutral pH and at room temperature with divalent cations and sulfated polysaccharides. Various techniques have been described for the isolation of VLDL, LDL, and HDL from large or small volumes of plasma. The precipitated lipoproteins may be further purified by reprecipitation or by ultracentrifugation. The details of all these methods have been described recently by *Burstein and Scholnick* [75].

In brief, 0.4 ml of 5% heparin and 0.5 ml of 1 M MnCl$_2$ are added to 10 ml serum. A precipitate appears rapidly and can be sedimented by centufugation at 6,000 g for 10 min. Another procedure involves the addition of 50 μl of 10% dextran sulfate and 0.5 ml of 1 M MnCl$_2$. VLDL and LDL are completely precipitated and could be removed by centrifugation. By proportionately changing the volume of reagents, the precipitation can be carried out in smaller or larger volumes of plasma [75, 76].

In both cases, the clear supernatant contains HDL while the precipitates contain VLDL and LDL; therefore, for any studies requiring the isolation of cholesterol in the two lipoproteins separately, VLDL have to be removed by some other method before precipitating the LDL. The VLDL are generally removed by preparative ultracentrifugation of the plasma. Alternatively, they can be selectively precipitated using appropriate concentrations of sodium lauryl sulfate and incubation at 35 °C [74]. HDL can also be precipitated by adding appropriate amounts of 10% dextran sulfate and 1 M MnCl$_2$ [76]. For SA of cholesterol, the precipitates may need to be washed once or twice with the solutions containing dextran sulfate and maganese chloride. For more detailed studies, the precipitates can be dissolved in appropriate solutions and purified either by reprecipitation or by ultracentrifugation [75].

Extraction and Purification of Cholesterol

All solvents used for extraction, etc., should be of reagent grade and should be redistilled if they are not of the highest grade. This is particularly important when large volumes of solvents are evaporated to yield lipid samples in small volumes for subsequent analysis. It is also desirable to test all solvents used in the laboratory for presence of residues (after their evaporation) by sensitive methods such as gas-liquid chromatography (GLC).

All glassware used in the laboratory should have either ground glass tapered joints or teflon stoppers. Stopcock grease should not be used in a laboratory where lipid analyses are performed routinely. Similarly, o-rings are undesirable in any apparatus used for lipid analysis unless they are made of teflon, etc.

In order to remove all lipids from plasma lipoproteins, it is necessary to break the lipid-protein bond by denaturing the proteins. A number of solvent systems have been used to extract lipids from plasma; however, the most common solvent system used is chloroform : methanol (2:1) introduced by *Folch et al.* [145, 146]. *Folch et al.* used this solvent system for extraction of lipids from tissues, and based on their work *Sperry and Brand* [444] recommended this solvent system for extraction of lipids from plasma. They recommended a solvent to sample ratio of 24:1 using 2:1 chloroform: methanol (v/v).

The plasma (or plasma lipoprotein) sample is first added to the volume of methanol and then half of the required volume of chloroform is added. The mixture is warmed in a water bath and then allowed to cool to room temperature. The remainder of the chloroform is then added to bring it up to the volume. The heating step can be omitted without any loss of extraction. The solution should be stirred for 5 min, mixed thoroughly, and filtered through a sintered glass funnel or a fast filter paper previously washed with chloroform methanol. The residue on the filter paper should be washed at least twice with 10-ml aliquots of chloroform:methanol to quantitatively collect the lipids in the filtrate. This method of extraction gives quantitative extraction of cholesterol and triglycerides [320].

Ethanol:ether (3:1 v/v) when used in excess of 20 volumes has been found to be a satisfactory mixture for extraction of neutral lipids [49, 62]. Neutral lipids can also be quantitatively extracted by hexane. To plasma (serum or lipoprotein fraction) ethanol and water are added to obtain 40% ethanol concentration and the lipids extracted with 3×5 volumes of hexane [384, 474]. Recently, *Cham and Knowles* [80] introduced a new method for complete delipidation of plasma using a mixture of butanol and di-isopropyl ether in 40:60 v/v ratio. To 1 volume of plasma, 2 volumes of the extraction mixture is added, and the tubes are fastened to a rotator to provide end-over-end rotation at 28–30 rpm, for 30 min, at the end of which they are centrifuged at 2,000 rpm for 2 min to separate aqueous and organic phase. The aqueous phase is then removed free of the organic phase. 20 volumes of isopropanol is used for the extraction of cholesterol and triglycerides, especially in procedures where estimation is carried out by autoanalyzer [45].

Extraction of Cholesterol from Tissues

Cholesterol from tissues such as liver, adipose tissue, brain, xanthoma, etc., is also extracted with chloroform:methanol (2:1). The sample is homogenized in a suitable tissue homogenizer with 25 volumes of chloroform: methanol (1:1 v/v). The solvent and tissue residue is transferred to a lipid-free fast grade filter paper, and the filtrate collected in a graduated cylinder. The tissue homogenizer and the residue is washed twice with 5 volumes of 1:1 chloroform:methanol. The filtrate is then brought to a final volume with chloroform so that the proportions of chloroform and methanol are 2:1 (v/v) and the ratios of solvent to tissue (1 g) is 50:1 [146, 320].

Extraction of cholesterol from RBC is complicated by the presence of hemoglobin which on denaturation retains large amounts of solvents and lipid in a matrix that is difficult to flush adequately. For RBC extraction, the cells are first added slowly to methanol. Drop-wise addition of cells to large volumes of methanol (10:1 solvent to sample ratio) results in a fine dispersion of precipitated hemoglobin provided the solution is kept stirred. Chloroform is then added to make the chloroform:methanol volume 2:1. It is filtered and processed in the same way as the extracts of plasma [320].

Saponification of Cholesterol in Plasma or Tissues

If the investigator is interested in only total cholesterol, plasma, bile or tissues can be subjected to saponification before extraction of cholesterol.

The plasma or bile sample (2–4 ml) is transferred to a 50-ml glass-stoppered centrifuge tube and 10 ml of methanolic KOH is added to obtain a final concentration of KOH 10% (v/v) and of methanol 70%. Tissues (up to 500 mg) after cutting into small pieces are also transferred to 50-ml glass-stoppered centrifuge tubes. 3 ml of distilled water is added and then 10 ml of methanolic KOH to obtain a KOH concentration of 20% w/v and methanol 70% (a known amount of radioactive cholesterol may be added to serve as an internal standard). The mixture is saponified at 70°C for 2 h, and the nonsaponifiable fraction is extracted with 20 ml of petroleum ether (PE) (BP 30–60°C) thrice and the extracts pooled, evaporated, and made into a known amount of solvent [269].

Purification of the Extracts

The chloroform methanol extracts of plasma or other tissues may contain appreciable quantities of non-lipid material. To remove these contaminants, wash the lipid extract by thoroughly mixing it with one fifth (0.2) its volume of either water or of 0.29% sodium chloride solution [146]. The mixture should be allowed to separate into clear phases either by standing or centrifugation. The upper phase is removed by siphoning as completely as possible without losing any of the lower phase. The lower phase and the remaining upper phase are made into a single phase by addition of some methanol. This washing procedure is adequate for the extracts containing cholesterol.

Dextran-gel column purification is another but less commonly nsed method whereby a lipid extract can be purified essentially free of all non-lipid components [287, 411, 512].

Storage

Total lipid extracts and purified lipid fractions can be stored for long periods without significant deterioration provided proper storage conditions and adequate precautions are observed. The samples should be stored at as low a temperature as possible but not above −20°C. The samples should not be dry and should be stored as solution in organic solvents. Containers should be flushed with nitrogen to remove as much oxygen as possible and should be stored in the dark. Samples can be stored in screw cap vials provided the caps are thoroughly cleaned and lined with teflon or polyethylene sealers. Caps with bonded paper liners or plastic liners should not be used. Similarly, corks, rubber stoppers or wax paper covering should never be used. Ground glass-stoppered glassware is good for storing lipid extracts provided the stopper fits well. The commercially available ground glass-stoppered glassware is not ground finely enough to provide an adequate seal for organic solvents. These seals can be made tighter by a brief regrinding of the stopper with glass-grinding compound (aluminum oxide, 800 grit size).

Storage of lipids should be done in solvents like hexane and chloroform. Hexane is quite adequate for storing cholesterol, triglycerides, and fatty acids. Methanol or ethanol are not good solvents to store free fatty acids since methyl or ethyl ethers may form on prolonged storage [32, 214, 320, 385].

Separation of Free and Esterified Cholesterol

Free cholesterol can be conveniently separated from esterified cholesterol and other plasma and tissue lipids by: (1) thin-layer chromatography (TLC); (2) column chromatography, and (3) digitonin precipitation.

Thin-Layer Chromatography

The speed and versatility of TLC and its ability to resolve compounds even with minimal differences in their chemical structure make it an especially valuable analytical tool. The technique is based on the principle of adsorption and partition chromatography, and some excellent reviews on its use for separation of lipids are available [354, 423, 445].

Preparation of Thin-Layer Plates

Borosilicate glass plates (20 × 20 cm) are thoroughly cleaned by first soaking them in dilute chromic acid-sulphuric acid mixture and then rinsing extensively with distilled water. The plates are dried in an oven and are coated with silica gel. Various preparations of the silica gel can be used, e.g. silica gel G, H, HR, etc. For analytical work, a silica gel layer of 250μm thickness is generally used. For preparative work, a thicker coating (up to 500 μm) is used in order to resolve larger quantities of material.

The required amount of silica gel is weighed in a 500-ml bottle with a ground-glass stopper, and distilled water is then added (generally) in a (silica gel:water) ratio of 1:2. The mixture is shaken thoroughly to obtain a uniform slurry. Any trapped air bubbles are removed from the slurry by tapping the bottle. The slurry is then poured into the reservoir of the spreader (in any one of many commercially available equipment), and the silica gel is spread by pulling the spreader evenly over the plates with a uniform smooth pull. Abrupt changes in speed produce nonuniform layers. Therefore, the plates should be properly leveled. It is preferable to use a spreading

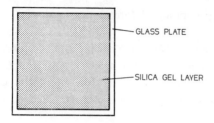

Fig. 3. Preparation of thin-layer plates for chromatography of lipids. After coating the plates with silica gel, the gel is removed from all four sides of the face of the glass plate to a depth of about 2 mm. This area is used for all subsequent handling of the plate.

assembly that levels the upper rather than the lower surface of the plate, so that variations in plate thickness will not affect the thickness of the coating. After the plates are coated, they are allowed to dry in the air for 10–15 min at room temperature and then placed in an oven at 110–120 °C for 20 min. The dry plates are then stored in a dessicator until needed. It is not always necessary to prepare the silica gel plates in one's own laboratory since a large variety of precoated plates are commercially available.

Washing the Thin-Layer Plates

When exposed to air, coated plates adsorb impurities from the air. Therefore, it is a good practice to wash the plates free of contamination by developing the plates in a mixture of chloroform:methanol:water (80:20:1). The solvent mixture and the impurities are allowed to run up to the top of the plate from where the impurities are removed by scraping away the silica gel along the upper border of the plate (fig. 3). The plates should be reactivated in an oven at 110–120 °C for 20 min before use.

The silica gel should be removed from all four sides of the face of the glass plate to a depth of about 2 mm, and all subsequent handling of the plates should be limited to the areas devoid of the gel (fig. 3).

Application of Sample

The lipid mixture dissolved in a suitable solvent is applied on the plate either as a long, thin, horizontal streak, or alternatively as a small round spot. It is best to confine the original application to as small an area as possible, and this often entails considerable practice in the use of micropipettes or microsyringes. An intact tip is necessary for proper applications. Therefore, the tips of micropipettes should be protected from chipping. Care must also be taken to prevent damage to the coating during application. When using microsyringes, allow a small bead of liquid to collect at the end of the needle before depositing it onto the surface of the plates without actually touching the coating with the needle. The syringes are particularly useful for application of the sample in a horizontal line. Several automatic and semi-automatic 'streaking' and 'spotting' devices are commercially available. Every effort should be made to make as narrow a line as possible. When larger volumes are involved, the sample should be applied repeatedly along the same line. To prevent excessive spreading of the sample, time should be allowed to completely dry the sample in between applications. The narrower the line of application the better the resolution.

Development of Thin-Layer Chromatogram

Immediately after the solvent containing the lipids is evaporated, the plate should be placed in the developing tank. It is worth emphasizing that lipids left dry and exposed to the air on thin-layer plates are easily oxidized [425]. Therefore, it is necessary to develop chromatograms and remove the lipids from thin-layer plates in as short a time as possible, and preferably with as little unnecessary exposure to room air as possible.

The plates are developed in special chromatography tanks generally made of glass and wide enough to hold 20 × 20 cm plates. All glass tanks can accommodate two plates and some with partitions can accommodate a much larger number. The walls of the jar should be lined with filter paper prewashed in organic solvents to remove impurities. About 100–150 ml of the solvent system is usually sufficient to cover the bottom of the TLC plate and the filter paper lining the insides of the tanks should be damp. Allow a few minutes for equilibration of the solvent with the atmosphere inside the tanks, and then transfer the TLC plates into tanks for development.

A number of different solvent systems are available for isolating FC and esterified cholesterol; each from other compounds in the lipid extracts. The most commonly used solvent system is hexane-diethyl ether-acetic acid (85:15:2 v/v/v) [157, 282]. This system gives a good resolution between CE, triglycerides, fatty acids, FC, and phospholipids. The 1,2-diglycerides tend to move close to FC and at times do not properly separate from cholesterol. However, they are generally present in trace amounts, and their elution with cholesterol will generally not affect the quantitation of cholesterol using methods which specifically estimate cholesterol. However, it might be important to isolate FC from possible contamination by diglycerides, as for example for determination of SA of FC after giving radioactive acetate which will also label diglycerides. Similarly, in other metabolic studies it may be necessary to purify cholesterol from other closely related sterols: these methods are described on page 21.

CE, as a class, are generally separated free of contamination from other lipids known to interfere with their evaluation. Their further separation into saturated, mono-, di-, and tetra-unsaturated esters could be done by the use of silica gel impregnated with silver nitrate [184, 305].

Collection of Lipids from Thin-Layer Plates

After development, the plates are taken out of the tank, the solvent is allowed to evaporate completely in a fume hood, and the location of lipids is visualized by any one of a number of different methods which may be destructive or nondestructive. The former generally involves charring of the compounds on TLC plates by any one of a number of reagents, most of which contain sulfuric acid [358, 386, 423]. A fine mist of the reagent is sprayed until the plate is uniformly covered. It is then transferred to an oven at 150–175 °C for 20 min to char the lipids. Methods have now been developed which allow quantitation of the lipids on TLC plates from the densitometric analysis of the charred material on thin-layer plates [118, 359, 360]. Such methods, however, have not yet been universally accepted.

Exposure of the plate to iodine vapor is a common nondestructive method for the visualization of lipids. Alternatively, the plates can be sprayed either with rhodamine 6G (0.001% solution in water) or with 2',7'-dichlorofluorescein (0.03% in 0.01 N NaOH), and the location of the lipids is visualized with short-wave UV light [283, 414].

The location of lipids is marked with a needle, keeping in mind that the concentration of lipids on the gel will have a normal bell-shaped distribution and the silica gel in the immediate vicinity of the visible spots may contain the lipid in amounts too small to be seen. Therefore, the boundaries of the lipid spots bands are marked with some 'safety margin'. The bands of silica gel containing the lipid can either be aspirated into special funnels with vacuum [161] or can be scraped with a razor blade and transferred into an eluting column or a sintered glass funnel. The free and esterified cholesterol are then eluted with large volumes of diethyl ether.

Column Chromatography

Free and esterified cholesterol can be separated from each other and from other lipids by column chromatography. Separation of CE by column chromatography was first described by *Borgström* [53, 54] and by *Fillerup and Mead* [141]. A systematic study for the separation of complex lipid mixtures by the use of silicic acid columns was carried out by *Hirsch and Ahrens* [203].

A number of variations and comprehensive schemes are now available for fractionating lipids by column chromatography. These modifications include refinements in the techniques of preparing columns, the use of different solvents for elution, and automation of the procedure [28, 319, 453].

Other adsorbents, such as Florisil [79] and lipophilic Sephadex [67, 128], have also been proposed, but the silica gel remains the mainstay of chromatography of lipids. The use of lipophilic Sephadex (LH20) has increased in recent years and shows considerable promise [81, 485].

The column chromatographic methods are best for large scale separation of lipids. They are, however, generally tedious and time-consuming, although they can be simplified and adapted for small-scale separations of free from esterified cholesterol [81].

Digitonin Precipitation

Isolation of FC can conveniently be done by precipitating it with digitonin. Since it is necessary to have a β-hydroxyl group at C3 for forming digitonide, CE cannot be precipitated by digitonin. *Windaus* [503, 504] was the first to show that FC forms precipitable digitonides. Since that time, digitonin has been used extensively to isolate β-hydroxy-sterols. *Schoenheimer* and co-workers [397–399] popularized the use of digitonin for isolating cholesterol from plasma and tissue. *Sperry and Webb* [443] and later *Sperry* [442] extended and standardized the conditions necessary to obtain excellent results.

For isolating FC from plasma (or serum), the sample of plasma is added slowly and with constant agitation in a volumetric flask containing 10–12 times its volume of acetone:ethanol (1:1 v/v). The mixture is then brought to a boil on a steam bath, cooled to room temperature, and the volume is adjusted to 25 ml by adding more acetone:alcohol for each ml of plasma. The mixture is thoroughly shaken and then filtered.

A known aliquot of the extract containing 0.5–4 mg of precipitable sterols is transferred to a centrifuge tube and the contents are made up to 4 ml by adding acetone:alcohol. 1 ml of 2% digitonin solution in 80% ethanol is added and then followed at once by the addition of 1 ml of water. The tubes are placed in a beaker which in turn is placed in a jar containing a small volume of the solvent mixture (acetone:ethanol:water 20:2.8:1.2) to saturate the atmosphere. The cover of the jar is tightly closed and the tubes are left overnight for complete precipitation of cholesterol digitonide. The following day, the walls of the tubes just above the surface of the liquid are scrubbed with a stirring rod to wet and loosen any precipitate which may be sticking to the walls of the tube. The tubes are centrifuged for 15 min at 2,800 rpm to pack down the precipitate. The supernatant is removed with a Pasteur pipette taking extreme care not to remove any precipitate. To wash the precipitate free of digitonin and other lipids, about 1.5 ml of 80% ethanol is added along the sides of the tube so as to wash down any adhering precipitate. The precipitate is then stirred into suspension and tubes are recentrifuged for 5 min and the supernatant solution is removed as before. The precipitate is washed twice more with 80% ethanol and three times with ether in the same way as above. The residual ether is removed by a gentle stream of nitrogen [442].

The FC can be estimated by gravimetric analysis of its digitonide or chemically by a number of methods [348, 518, 527]. If the cholesterol is to be determined gravimetrically, then the tubes used for precipitation should be preweighed. Before reweighing, however, the digitonide should be dried either overnight in vacuo over Drierite or in an oven at 110 °C for 1 h. The amount of cholesterol is determined by dividing the weight of digitonide by 4.18 [442].

Parekh et al. [350] have recently simplified the precipitation of plasma cholesterol with digitonin. In their method, cholesterol is precipitated from the isopropanol extract of the plasma using 1% digitonin (in 50% ethanol) solution. For the precipitation of the cholesterol digitonide, it is necessary to keep the tubes in the refrigerator at 4 °C for 30 min. The tubes are centrifuged at a high speed for 10 min, the supernatant discarded, and the precipitate is washed twice with acetone.

If the sample is radioactive, the digitonide can be dissolved in a small volume of methanol and the radioactivity counted in a liquid scintillation spectrometer after adding an appropriate scintillation mixture.

To isolate cholesterol from its digitonide, the precipitate is dissolved completely in a small volume of pyridine (0.3–0.5 ml). 3 ml of ether is added and the mixture thoroughly stirred. The tube is centrifuged for 5 min at 2,800 rpm and the supernatant containing cholesterol is transferred to another tube. The precipitate is washed three times with ether and the washings pooled. Ether is then removed under nitrogen and pyridine is removed by leaving the tube over H_2SO_4 in vacuo overnight. The free cholesterol is then dissolved in an appropriate solvent for estimation [442].

For isolating tissue cholesterol, the lipids should first be extracted with chloroform:methanol (2:1) as described earlier and the lipids picked up in acetone:alcohol (1:1). The digitonin precipitation is then carried out as described above for plasma or serum, making sure that the quantities of digitonin added are well in excess of those required for equimolar reaction.

Purification of Cholesterol

Cholesterol in various tissues, including plasma, is usually accompanied by its derivative cholestanol (dihydrocholesterol) or its precursors such as Δ^7-cholestenol (lathosterol), 7-dehydrocholesterol and desmosterol (fig. 1). It may also be contaminated with certain hydroxylated sterols produced by autooxidation on exposure to air or light. Normally, these sterols are present only in traces; therefore, it is not usually necessary to purify plasma cholesterol before its estimation. Cholesterol used as a standard, however, must be purified. Similarly, it may be necessary to purify cholesterol before estimating its radioactivity in certain metabolic studies.

Cholesterol can be purified by treatment with bromine in ether. Cholesterol is converted to insoluble $5\alpha,6\beta$-dibromide from which cholesterol can be regenerated by treatment of pure dibromide with zinc dust or acetic acid or sodium iodide. The contaminants are left in the mother liquor [138, 397]. An alternative method of purification involves crystallization of cholesterol from acetic acid. Cholesterol is stirred with boiling acetic acid until dissolved and then rapidly cooled in ice. Cholesterol separates as a complex which loses acetic acid on drying at 90 °C. This also serves to remove cholestanol and Δ^7-cholestenol effectively [137]. However, the dibromide method yields a material of higher molar absorptivity than that obtained by ethanol or acetic acid recrystallization [365, 499]. *Radin and Gramza* [365] recommended that molar absorptivities as produced by the Liebermann-Burchard (L-B) reaction (1,750±30) and by the iron salt-sulphuric acid procedure (11,500±100) can be used as a guide to the purity of a cholesterol preparation along with a melting point which was found to be 149.0–150.0 °C by *Fieser* [137, 138].

When cholesterol is recrystallized from moist solvents, it separates as a monohydrate. In order to remove water of crystallization, this material should be heated in an oven at 90 °C (not higher) for 2 h or in a vacuum oven at a lower temperature [476].

Purification of Cholesterol by TLC

Cholesterol can also be purified by TLC, and this method is especially suitable when only microgram amounts have to be purified. Purification cannot be done on usual adsorbents, and recourse to argentation TLC and reverse-phase TLC is necessary.

Argentation TLC

In argentation TLC, silica gel plates are prepared either by incorporating silver nitrate (anywhere between 6 and 12%) directly into the gel before making the plates or by spraying the prepared plates with 12–25% of AgNO₃ before activation [19, 230, 478]. One of the better methods for separation of cholesterol from accompanying sterols using argentation TLC has been described by *Daly* [95].

Aluminum oxide (type E) plates (0.25–0.5 mm) are prepared and after drying sprayed uniformly with 25% AgNO₃. The plates are activated at 120 °C for 20 min before use. The sterol mixture along with the standards is applied in a small narrow band and the plates are developed in chloroform. Separation obtained is shown diagramatically in figure 4. Although 20 × 20 cm plates can be used, separation is much better on a 40-cm plate. Cholestanol and Δ7-cholestenol do not always separate from each other. Their separation could be achieved by reverse-phase chromatography.

Reverse-Phase TLC

De Souza and Nes [111] described a reverse-phase TLC in which paraffin oil was used as the stationary phase and aqueous acetone saturated with paraffin as the mobile phase. This system not only separates closely related C_{27} sterols, but also closely related C_{28} and C_{29} sterols such as phyto sterols. The system is especially useful to purify fecal cholesterol which is usually contaminated with dietary plant sterols such as campesterol (C_{28}), β-sitosterol (C_{29}), and stigmasterol (C_{29}). Only a small amount of the sterol mixture (up to about 500 µg) can be separated using plates of 0.5 mm thickness by this method.

About 300 ml of acetone:water 4:1 is shaken in a separatory funnel with 30 ml of paraffin oil. The mixture is kept for 18 h at 24–25 °C. The two layers are then separated. The paraffin oil layer (lower phase) is diluted with PE (BP 30–60 °C) to a 5% solution. This solution is used for impregnation procedure. Glass plates 20 × 20 cm are coated with water:kieselguhr G (2:1). After drying, the plates are activated at 110 °C for 1 h, cooled to room temperature and impregnated with 5% paraffin solution by carefully introducing

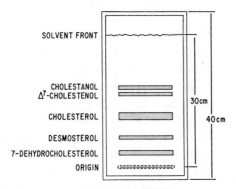

Fig. 4. TLC separation of cholesterol from other closely related C_{27} steroids present in animal tissues. The extra long glass plates (20 × 40 cm) are coated with aluminium oxide-silver nitrate and are developed in chloroform.

the plates into a tank filled with the solution. After 1 min, the plates are removed, held upside down for a few seconds, then kept at room temperature on a horizontal surface for 30 min. Recently, *Tint and Salen* [475] modified the method in that they used 5% solution of paraffin oil in PE without equilibration of paraffin oil with acetone:water. Impregnation is done by allowing the paraffin oil solution to migrate to the top of the plate and the plates used as soon as petroleum ether is evaporated.

About 100 ml of the solvent system (acetone:water [4:1 v/v]) is placed in a chromatographic jar lined with filter paper on three sides. The atmosphere in the tank is equilibrated at room temperature for at least 3 h. After spotting the sterol mixtures and the standards, the plates are developed up to a height of about 15 cm. The plates are removed, dried, and sterol bands are visualized by spraying lightly with a half saturated aqueous solution of rhodamine G. The kieselguhr containing the sterol is eluted first with ethyl ether, then with hexane, and finally with a 1:1 mixture of the two. This sequence has been found to give maximal recovery of the sterols [475]. However, paraffin is also eluted with the solvents used. To remove paraffin oil, the sterols are rechromatographed on kieselguhr G plates without paraffin oil and developed twice in *n*-heptane. The oil migrates with the solvent front leaving the sterol band behind [475].

For complete purification of cholesterol from other sterols, including plant sterols, both argentation TLC and 2–3 repetitions of reverse-phase chromatography may be required.

Separation of Individual CE

The separation of CE as a class from other lipid classes can be achieved by column or TLC as described earlier. Both the sterol content and the fatty acid composition can be estimated with or without hydrolysis of CE [254, 255]. The fatty acids can be determined by GLC and the sterol by GLC or other chemical methods. However, in some metabolic studies specifically involving the distribution of radioactivity in various classes of CE, one may need to fractionate individual CE before their quantitation. This can be achieved by TLC on silica gel G impregnated with silver nitrate. This method produces rapid and wide separation of CE differing in the number of double bonds in the fatty acid moiety. Different amounts of silver nitrate and different solvent systems have been employed [151, 165, 305]. By carrying out two successive chromatographies in two solvent systems, many groups of CE from saturated to hexaunsaturated may each be isolated. One such method is described below. The plates are first developed with hexane: diethylether:acetic acid (70:29:1). In this solvent systemt tri-, tetra-, and pentaunsaturated esters separate from one another. The hexaunsaturated esters remain at the origin, and the saturated, monounsaturated and di-unsaturated esters move to the top with the solvent front. The esters at the solvent front are eluted from the gel and replated on $AgNO_3$ plates and chromatographed in benzene:hexane (60:40). In this system, saturated, monounsaturated, and diunsaturated CE are separated from one another [151]. Further separation of CE with some degree of unsaturation or of different saturated esters, from each other, if desired, can then be achieved by reverse-phase chromatography [252, 257]. It should be noted that un-saturated esters are relatively difficult to elute from the gel. All CE, however, can be completely eluted from the gel with warm benzene:ether (1:1 v/v) [151, 164].

Estimation of Cholesterol

A great variety of methods are available for the estimation of total, FC and esterified cholesterol in the lipid extracts. Critical reviews on most of these methods have been published [476, 517]. Cholesterol can be estimated by: (1) gravimetric method; (2) colorimetric methods; (3) densitometric methods; (4) fluorometric methods; (5) gas chromatographic methods; (6) enzymatic methods, and (7) isotope derivative method.

Gravimetric Method

The gravimetric method was the earliest method used to measure cholesterol. *Windaus* showed that digitonin can precipitate cholesterol in 1:1 molecular complex. The weight of the sterol digitonide is 4.18 times that of cholesterol, i.e. 1 mg cholesterol when precipitated as cholesterol digitonide will weigh 4.18 mg. Cholesterol in CE can be determined by the same method after its saponification to free cholesterol. The method, however, is not specific since all the sterols containing the hydroxyl group at the 3β position are precipitated by digitonin. Furthermore, conditions for precipitation and washing the complex free of digitonin are of critical importance [442].

Wood and Weizel [510] reported a gravimetric method which involved separation of FC and esterified cholesterol by TLC and their elution in preweighed vials. After evaporation of the solvents, the vials are reweighed to obtain the amounts of FC and esterified cholesterol. The applicability of this method, however, is limited to samples containing relatively large quantities of pure cholesterol, free of all contaminants.

Colorimetric Methods

Cholesterol and other related sterols when treated with various acid reagents give intense color depending upon the type of acid used and concentration of the sterol. This reaction forms the basis of many colorimetric methods. Two major advantages of this approach are: (a) small quantities ($\approx 0.5{-}1$ μg) of cholesterol can be determined, and (b) the test is specific for cholesterol or cholesterol-like compounds so that their concentration can be determined in the presence of other lipids. Usually, the concentrations of other sterols in plasma or tissue extracts are small so that their contributions to the color reaction can generally be ignored. However, in certain metabolic studies, it may be necessary to purify cholesterol before its estimation.

Direct determination of cholesterol in plasma or tissue extracts may also be affected by other substances, e.g. bilirubin. It is therefore important that the interfering substances are removed as far as possible before development of the color.

Color reagents do not necessarily give identical color intensity for identical amounts of cholesterol present in either free or the esterified form. For example, it was shown by *Webster* [493, 494] that the L-B reaction gives more color with CE than with FC. Therefore, if only FC is used as a standard, total cholesterol and CE may be overestimated. A few of the commonly used methods are described below.

Liebermann-Burchard Method

Among the many color reactions for cholesterol, the L-B procedure is perhaps the most widely used. The reaction was described initially by *Liebermann* [262] in 1885 and applied to cholesterol analysis by *Burchard* [73]. Chloroform was used as solvent in early studies, but the L-B procedure as performed today is carried out in acetic acid, sulfuric acid and acetic anhydride. Although most recent modifications have used the same three reagents, there are almost as many variations in their use as there are investigators. *Abell*'s procedure [2] is considered to be the most accurate and reliable and has been used as a standard for other methods. This method is therefore described in detail.

Preparation of Reagent. 20 volumes of acetic anhydride are chilled to a temperature lower than 10 °C and 1 volume of concentrated sulfuric acid is added, mixed, and kept cold for 9 min. 10 volumes of glacial acetic acid are then added and the mixture is warmed to room temperature. The reagent is prepared just prior to use.

Procedure. 0.5 ml plasma sample is pipetted into a 25-ml glass-stoppered centrifuge tube and 5 ml of freshly prepared alcoholic potassium hydroxide (prepared by adding 6 ml of 33% KOH to 94 ml absolute ethanol) is added. After thorough mixing, the tube is incubated in a water bath at 37–40 °C for 55 min and then cooled to room temperature. 10 ml of PE (BP 68 °C) is added and mixed, followed by 5 ml of water and thorough mixing again for 1 min in a mechanical mixer. The tube is then centrifuged at slow speed for 5 min to separate the phases. A suitable aliquot (containing between 0.15 and 0.60 mg of cholesterol) of the upper PE phase is transferred to another tube and the solvent is evaporated to dryness under a gentle stream of air or nitrogen.

The tube containing the dry residue is kept in a water bath at 25 °C and 6 ml of freshly prepared L-B reagent is added taking care to wash down the entire inner surface of the tube with the reagent. The contents of the tube are mixed well and then returned to the bath. The optical density of the blue green color is read against the blank in a photoelectric colorimeter at 620 nm 30–35 min after the reagent is added.

One of the disadvantages of this method is the unstability of the color. Earlier preparations of L-B reagents were unstable; however, in recent years, more stable versions of the L-B reagent have been prepared [217, 234, 321], and the procedure has been modified to decrease the time and skill necessary for its performance. The reaction is complex and is affected by many variables, e. g. the solvent employed to dissolve cholesterol, the water, the time of reaction, the temperature, the wavelength at which the color is measured, the presence of interfering substances such as bilirubin, the (unreacted) digitonin and whether the cholesterol is esterified or free. The conditions of assay must therefore be standardized and rigidly adhered to [476, 493, 494, 517].

A variant of L-B method was introduced by *Pearson et al.* [353]. The use of *p*-toluene sulfonic acid (P-TSA) instead of L-B reagent was shown to result in a more stable color after its development. Also, FC and esterified cholesterol produced the same intensity of color, thereby eliminating the need for saponification. A number of modifications of this modification have also been reported [188, 511, 528].

Methods Utilizing Iron Salts and Sulphuric Acid

These reagents were first used to determine the amounts of cholesterol by *Zlatkis et al.* [527]. The reaction is carried out in acetic acid and sulfuric acid in the presence of iron salts. $Fe(^{+++})$ is added to obtain the desired color which is several times more intense than that obtained by the L-B or P-TSA reagent systems. This makes these methods ideally suited for micro and ultramicro samples. The color is also reasonably stable and is not sensitive to light. The intensity of color with FC is the same as that with esterified cholesterol, and therefore saponification of CE is not necessary. Cholesterol digitonide also gives the same color as the FC and the traces of free digitonin do not interfere. However, hemoglobin and bilirubin do interfere somewhat with the color reaction.

Many modifications of the method generally involving the use of different $Fe(^{+++})$ salts have been described. Thus, ferric chloride, ferric sulphate, ferric ammonium chloride, and ferric perchlorate have all been used [383, 403, 513, 519]. The original reagent (ferric chloride in sulfuric acid) was not stable, but a dilute solution of ferric chloride in acetic acid has been found to be stable for at least a month at room temperature.

The $FeCl_3$-acetic acid reagent is added to the test material followed by the addition of sulfuric acid. Cholesterol gives a purple color which is read at 560 nm. One of the most important sources of error in the iron salt-sulphuric acid methods is improper mixing after adding the sulphuric acid. A standardized rapid method of mixing which produces maximum temperature must be used. Care should be taken not to produce bubbles which can cause large errors.

A recent variation of the method was proposed by *Parekh and Jung* [348] for direct estimation of cholesterol in plasma. They employed ferric acetate, uranium acetate, sulfuric acid and ferrous sulfate reagents. The ferric acetate and uranium acetate precipitate and remove bilirubin (as biliverdin) and proteins, clear the serum, and serve to extract total cholesterol without the need of solvents. This extract when mixed with the sulfate reagent yields a purple color with an absorption maximum at 560 nm. The maximum intensity of color develops in 15 min and is stable for at least 1 h. By reducing the volumes, *Parekh and Creno* [349] applied this method for estimating cholesterol in submicroliter volumes of biological fluids and for microgram amounts of frozen-dried tissues containing 0.05–3 μg of cholesterol.

In 1973, *Rudel and Morris* [387] introduced another method using O-phthalaldehyde reagent originally described by *Zlatkis and Zak* [526]. The method is three times more sensitive than the $FeCl_3$ method. A 50-mg/dl solution of O-phthalaldehyde in glacial acetic acid is prepared and 2 ml of this reagent is added to the sample and mixed thoroughly. After 10 min, 1 ml of concentrated sulfuric acid is carefully added by allowing it to run down the sides of the tubes. The solutions are then immediately mixed and the color is read at 550 nm, 20 min after the addition of concentrated sulfuric acid. The advantages of this method are that: (a) the reagent is easy to prepare; (b) the development of color is immediate and complete, and (c) the color is stable and insensitive to light. The assay is relatively specific for cholesterol. Cholestanol, the sterol which is present in highest concentration in most tissue extracts, does not give significant absorption at 550 nm.

Densitometric Methods

A useful procedure for measuring the mass of lipids resolved by TLC is photodensitometric scanning. The method involves the measurement of transmitted light with special photodensitometric apparatus. The instrument is adjusted to 100% transmission when the shutter in front of the photocell is closed. The passage of each spot over the slit gives a peak of optical density values. The area under the peak gives a linear relationship (which passes through the origin) with the amount of the sample expressed in terms of its carbon content of charred spots. For optimum accuracy, standards must be chromatographed on the same plates using concentrations similar to that of the samples being assayed.

Many techniques have been employed to char the lipids on developed chromatograms. Basically, it involves heating the plate at a high temperature in the presence of sulfuric acid, e.g. spraying the plate with an aqueous solution of 70% sulfuric acid saturated with potassium dichromate and heating the plate at 180 °C for 25 min.

Analysis may also be performed by determination of color spots given in a chromogenic reaction by use of specific filters. Although the method has potential usefulness, a lot of technological and methodological difficulties have yet to be resolved. Two mayor problems are nonuniform layers of adsorbents and nonuniform spraying and charring [243, 285, 360].

Fluorometric Methods

Cholesterol can be estimated by fluorometric methods [9, 52, 520]. They are generally based on modification of *Tschugaeff*'s [479] reaction. Fluorometric methods are very sensitive and therefore useful in estimating ultramicro levels. However, they are not in common use.

Gas-Liquid Chromatography

GLC is one of the most valuable techniques used in research laboratories for a number of years. In recent years, its use in clinical laboratories is also increasing. Although comprehensive methods have recently been proposed for quantitating free as well as esterified cholesterol in the same mixture [221, 254, 255], most columns used in the GLC are able only to resolve the free sterols and not their esters. Therefore, it is generally necessary to hydrolyze the esters before estimating the sterols by GLC. If total cholesterol (after saponification of the extract), and FC in extract (without saponification) are determined by GLC, the amounts of CE can be determined from the difference.

Alcoholic potassium hydroxide is often used for saponification of CE [46, 120, 193]. An inadvertent injection of KOH (alkaline aqueous phase), however, can adversely affect column performance. *MacGee et al.* [276] therefore suggested that tetramethylammonium hydroxide (TMH) be used as a saponifying agent since it has no adverse effects on column performance. *Ishikawa et al.* [223] recently developed a GLC method which can be used for quantitative analysis of cholesterol in as low as 5–20 μl of plasma. Their method is described below.

Tetramethylammonium hydroxide-isopropanol (TMH-i) solution is prepared by diluting 20 mg of 5α-cholestane (dissolved in 2 ml of diethylether) and 25 ml of TMH (24% in methanol) to 100 ml with isopropanol. 100 μl of TMH-i solution is placed in a 3-ml glass-stoppered conical centrifuge tube and 20 μl plasma samples is then added, tube stoppered and mixed on a vortex mixer for 10 sec. The tube is then heated in a heating block at 80 °C for 15 min. After cooling, 50 μl of solution containing 1 part of tetrachlorethylene and 3 parts of methylbutyrate is added to the tube and the contents thoroughly mixed, again following the addition of 200 μl of distilled water. The contents are mixed vigorously again. It is then centrifuged at 2,000–2,500 rpm for 10 min. 0.5–1 μl of the clear lower phase (tetrachloroethylene) is then injected into the gas chromatograph equipped with flame ionization detectors.

A silanized glass column (1.8 m × 2 mm [ID]) packed with 3% OV-17 on 100–200 mesh gas chrom Q is used. Column temperature is maintained at 260 °C, injection port temperature 290 °C and detector temperature at 300 °C. Nitrogen-carrier gas is maintained at a flow rate 50 ml/min, hydrogen 30 ml/min, and nitrogen:oxygen (60:40%) is used at a flow rate of 300 ml/min.

To minimize the effects of adsorption of cholesterol by solid support, 2 μl of cholesterol solution (3 mg/ml) is used to prime the column prior to the injection of sample.

For estimating FC, the serum sample is extracted after addition of a known amount of internal standard. Extraction could be carried out by a number of different procedures described elsewhere. An aliquot from the known volume of extract is then analyzed by GLC as described above.

A number of different internal standards, column packings, and operational conditions have been used by different investigators. Thus, 5α-cholestane, β-sitosterol, stigmasterol, cholesteryl acetate, 11-ketoprogesterone have all been used as internal standards [193, 221, 276, 454]. Use of internal standards facilitates quantitation by permitting correction of data for methodological losses. When using the internal standard, the exact amount of sample injected into the gas chromatograph is not important. A number of column packings such as 3% OV-17, 3.8% SE-30, 1% DC 560, SP-2250, etc. coated on different adsorbents, have been used. Operative conditions also vary, e. g. temperatures of column have ranged from 220 to 300 °C. The injection port and detector temperatures are generally about 20–25 °C higher than the column temperature. Some investigators have prepared trimethyl silyl ethers of cholesterol before subjecting them to analysis by GLC.

Enzymatic Methods

There is a surge of interest in the development of enzymatic methods for the determination of cholesterol. Although enzyme kits are now commercially available, it would be some time before their place in research or clinical laboratory is firmly established. *Flegg* [143] and *Richmond* [372] were first to apply the enzymatic method for the assay of cholesterol in saponified serum. Later, *Allain et al.* [11] and *Tarbutton and Gunter* [471] developed complete enzymatic procedures for estimating plasma FC and total cholesterol. These methods are based on the following principles.

CE are hydrolyzed to FC by CE hydrolase (EC 3.1.13). The FC produced is then oxidized by cholesterol oxidase (EC 1.1.3.6) to cholest-4-en-3-one with simultaneous production of hydrogen peroxide (H_2O_2).

$$CE \xrightarrow{\text{CE hydrolase}} FC + \text{fatty acids,}$$

$$FC \xrightarrow{\text{chol. oxidase}} \text{cholestenone} + H_2O_2.$$

The released hydrogen peroxide can be estimated by a number of different methods. Thus, it is measured colorimetrically by oxidation of methanol to formaledhyde in the presence of catalase (EC 1.11.1.6). The formaldehyde reacts with ammonium ions and acetylacetone to form 3,5-diacetyl-1,4-dihydrolutidine, the extinction coefficient of which is then measured at 405 nm [351, 374, 376, 377], or by oxidative coupling of 4-amino-antipyrine and phenol in the presence of peroxidase (EC 1.11.1.7). The chromogen formed is measured at 500 nm [11, 304]. Instead of 4-amino-antipyrine and phenol, *O*-dianisidine can also be used. The color developed is measured at 450 nm [471]. Catalase coupled with aldehyde dehydrogenase (aldehyde: NAD[P] oxidoreductase [EC 1.2.15]) has also been used to measure the H_2O_2 [186]. The advantage of the last method over comparable methods are: the reaction is completed in a few minutes and the use of NAD^+ or $NADP^+$ permits the direct calculation of the substrate concentration from the absorbance value without reference to a standard solution.

Recently, a number of new modifications of the enzymatic determination of cholesterol have been published [117, 256, 302, 336]. These methods are based on measuring the release of peroxide itself as the rate of oxygen uptake during the oxidation of cholesterol by cholesterol oxidase. *Dietschy et al.* [117] reported the use of the oxygen electrode in a modified glucose analyzer for the enzymatic measurement of FC and esterified cholesterol levels in plasma lipoproteins and subcellular fractions of cells. Their assay procedure is described below.

Buffer and Enzyme Preparation. 400 mM potassium phosphate buffer (pH 7.5) and containing Triton X-100 (0.1%) is prepared and equilibrated with atmospheric oxygen at 37°C at least overnight before use. CE hydrolase solution is prepared fresh before use, by dissolving 100 mg of powdered enzyme (0.23 U/mg) in 0.4 ml of phosphate buffer by vigorous mixing in a

Vortex mixer. Contaminating FC is eliminated by adding 10–25 μl of cholesterol oxidase and incubating the mixture at 37 °C for 10–15 min. The mixture is stored in ice during use. Cholesterol oxidase solution at a concentration of 1 g/l (20 U/mg) is used. This solution is also prepared in a phosphate buffer.

Instrument. A standard glucose analyzer with two modifications is used for measuring the rate of oxygen uptake. The variable resistor controlling cabinet temperature is adjusted to give a mean temperature of 37 °C and the magnetic stirring turbine in the sample cup is replaced with a small 2 × 7 mm teflon-coated magnetic stirring bar to reduce the degree of stirring in the chamber. The amplified signal output from the electrode is fed to a chart recorder and is usually set to operate at 0.2 in/min using a 100-mV scale.

Assay Procedure. The sample cup of glucose analyzer is filled with 2.0 ml of 400 mM phosphate buffer (pH 7.50) containing 0.1% Triton X-100 (v/v). 10 μl of cholesterol oxidase alone (for measuring FC) or in combination of 20 μl CE hydrolase (for measuring total cholesterol) is added to the buffer solution followed by 10–20 μl of human plasma. The size of the sample depends on the type of biological fluid or tissue, e.g. plasma, bile or tissue. A standard cholesterol curve is run with each set of samples.

After the maximal level of oxygen utilization is reached, the height of each peak is compared to a standard cholesterol curve to obtain the concentration of cholesterol in the sample.

The enzymatic methods are rapid, reproducible, sensitive, and simple. They can be adapted for measuring sterol levels in a variety of biological preparations. All the reagents may be formulated into a one-step liquid reactive system so that analysis is conducted by simply adding reagents to the serum, incubating and reading. The only disadvantage of this method is that the reaction is not specific for cholesterol alone and other closely related sterols, e.g. cholestanol, lathosterol, 7-dehydrocholesterol are also oxidized by the enzyme [68, 310]. However, their quantities in plasma are negligible compared to cholesterol, and their rate of oxidation is very slow so that they are unlikely to affect the results significantly.

Isotope Derivative Method

Nicolau et al. [332] developed a method called the isotope derivative method for microdetermination of FC or total cholesterol. The method is sensitive to 0.1 nmol of cholesterol and is based on the conversion of cholesterol into its acetate by use of ³H-labeled acetic anhydride of known specific radioactivity.

In this procedure, the FC or total cholesterol extract is reacted with [³H]-acetic anhydride in pyridine. The [³H]-acetoxycholesterol is separated by TLC and the radioactivity assayed by scintillation counting. Since acetylation of cholesterol is quantitative, the amount of cholesterol is given by:

$$\frac{\text{Total radioactivity of [³H] acetoxycholesterol}}{\text{SA of [³H] acetic anhydride}}.$$

The method is rapid, extremely sensitive and especially suitable for quantitation of cholesterol from tissue cells [332].

Chapter III. Radioisotopes in Use for the Study of Cholesterol Metabolism

Cholesterol or its precursors labeled with ^{14}C or ^{3}H are frequently used in studies on cholesterol metabolism. Cholesterol labeled with ^{14}C in 4 and 26 carbon position and with ^{3}H in 1–2α and 7α are commercially available. Selection of isotope depends upon the purpose of the study.

Cholesterol-26-^{14}C and 7α ^{3}H cannot be used for the metabolic studies (e.g. cholesterol balance) which may involve quantitation of fecal bile acids by isotopic methods. When cholesterol is converted to bile acids, the labels 26-^{14}C and 7α ^{3}H are lost from the steroid molecule. Therefore, for such studies cholesterol-4-^{14}C and cholesterol-1α-2$\alpha$$^{3}H$ may be used. The distribution of radioactive atoms in cholesterol from biosynthetic incorporation of labeled precursors, e.g. acetate and mevalonate (fig. 5, 6) is such that some of the radioactive atoms are lost during its conversion to bile acids. Mevalonic acid-1-^{14}C cannot be used since the ^{14}C of 1 position is lost during its conversion to cholesterol.

Cholic acid, chenodeoxycholic acid, deoxycholic acid, and lithocholic acid labeled with ^{14}C and ^{3}H are other compounds used in the study of cholesterol metabolism. In some studies, CE labeled in fatty acids and plant sterols such as β-sitosterol ^{14}C or ^{3}H are used.

Most of these isotopes are available from several radiochemical manufacturers. The manufacturers will generally supply information on radiochemical purity; the investigator must also check each new lot before use. Both chemical and radiopurity must be established independently of each other. Merely because a given sample is greater than 99% pure chemically is no assurance that this also holds true for its radiopurity and vice versa. For example, a preparation of iodinated lipids having a chemical purity of >95% when examined for radiopurity showed that less than 60% of the radioactivity was present with iodinated lipids. Similarly, when a sample of (2,4-^{3}H) cholic acid with greater than 98% radiopurity was subjected to TLC, it was found that the desired 3α-hydroxy compound was contaminated by 3β-hydroxy epimer formed in the tritiation procedure. Only about 85% of the total radioactivity was found in the 3α-hydroxy band [346]. The use of

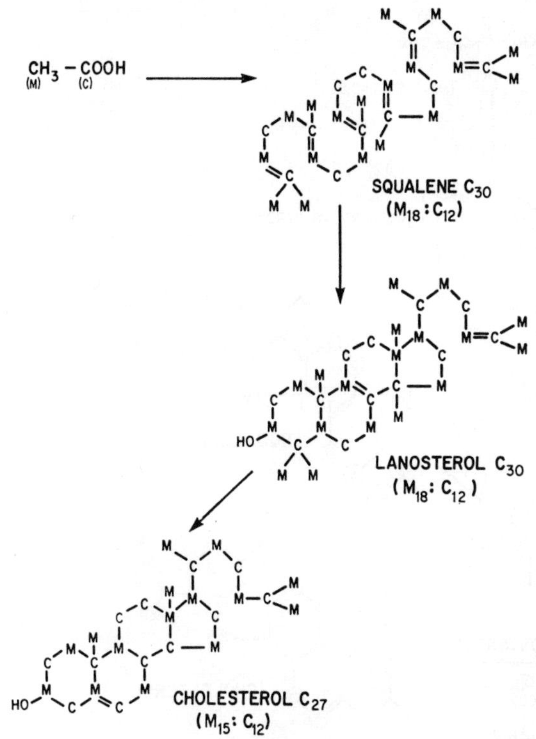

Fig. 5. Sites of incorporation of methyl (M) and carboxyl (C) carbon atoms of acetate into squalene, lanosterol, and cholesterol.

such materials for metabolic studies would obviously be a frustrating experience.

The isotopes should be checked for chemical and radiopurity by a number of different methods; most common being TLC alone or in combination with GLC. Chemicals have a limited shelf-life and it may vary with the condition of storage and handling. So far as possible, such degradation should be prevented by using reduced temperatures, proper solvents, and an environment free of oxygen. The decomposition caused by a higher concentration of radioactivity in a small sample is a real phenomenon and every effort should be directed to minimize this added problem. Testing the purity and purification should be made just before the experiments in order to avoid further decomposition during storage [309].

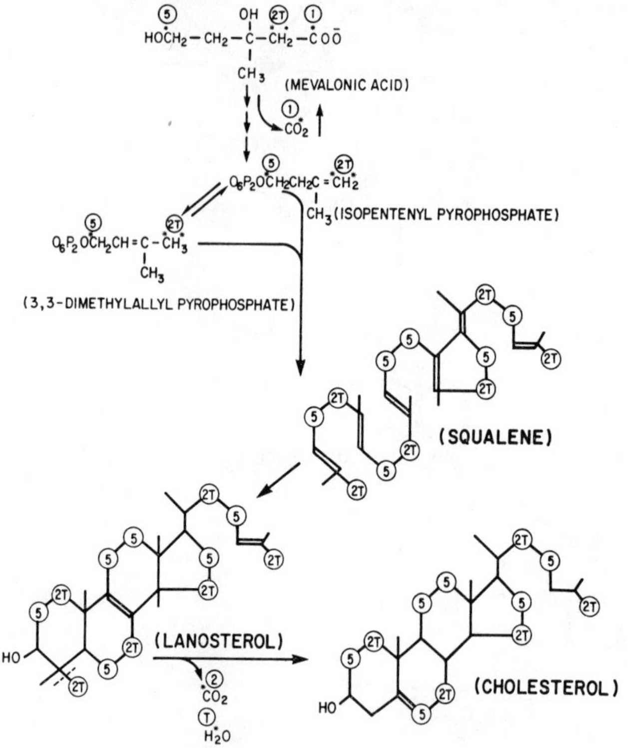

Fig. 6. Sites of incorporation of carbons 1, 2, and 5 and of hydrogen at position 2 of mevalonic acid into squalene, lanosterol, and cholesterol during their biosynthesis.

Purification of Isotopes

Isotopes of both cholesterol and bile acids are generally supplied as solutions in benzene and should be kept at room temperature until opened. The benzene should be evaporated under nitrogen and the material should be immediately redissolved in appropriate solvent. Isotopes should be obtained a few days in advance of the planned study, and they should not be allowed to remain as dry solids at room temperature for more than a few hours. Similarly, exposure to strong sunlight should be avoided.

Radiochemical Purity of Cholesterol

After the benzene has been evaporated, a little ethanol is added and the material is transferred into a volumetric flask. A small aliquot (10–20 μl) is transferred to a vial and a few milligrams of chemically pure cholesterol is added as a carrier to the vial. The sample dissolved in chloroform is quantitatively transferred onto a thin-layer plate coated with silica gel G (previously washed in methanol:ether, 1:4, and reactivated before use) and chromatographed using an appropriate solvent system. A number of different solvent systems can be used. One of the most commonly used systems is ethyl ether:heptane (55:45) [178]. Other solvent systems such as acetone: benzene (1:9), cyclohexane:ethylacetate (6:4), and benzene:ethyl acetate (5:1) are also used [19, 29]. After developing the chromatogram, the position of the carrier cholesterol is located by exposing the plate to iodine vapors. The zone of cholesterol is outlined with a needle, and the rest of the plate is divided from origin to solvent front into zones of equal width. The bands are then scraped, eluted, and the radioactivity determined. A strip scanner may also be used. Most of the recovered radioactivity should have mobility corresponding to the carrier cholesterol. If necessary, the sample should be purified by preparative TLC before use. Cholestanol is a common contaminant of cholesterol. It can be removed by TLC on silica gel G impregnated with silver nitrate and developing the chromatogram in chloroform:acetone (98:2) [478]. Other methods for purification of cholesterol are discussed on page 21.

Radiochemical Purity of Bile Acids

Procedures are generally identical to those listed above for cholesterol, except that bile acids are used as carriers. The samples are applied quantitatively to silica gel G 'plates'. They are then developed in a solvent system which separates the desired bile acids. Various solvent systems which could be used are listed in table I.

Radiochemical Purity of Acetate and Mevalonate

Radioactive acetic acid could be purified by steam distillation and its purity checked by GLC equipped with radioactivity counter [259, 371].

The radiochemical purity of mevalonic acid could be checked by paper chromatography in n-butanol:formic acid:water (70:30:120) or ethanol: 15 N NH_4OH:H_2O (8:1:1) or on silica gel G using benzene:acetone (1:1) [142, 404, 405].

It can be purified by preparing dibenzylethylenediamine salts and then its repeated extraction with ether [418]. However, commercially available preparations of radioacetate and mevalonate are generally quite satisfactory.

Table I. Colors given by different spray reagents with bile acids

Spray reagent	Cholic acid	Chenodeoxycholic acid	Deoxycholic acid	Lithocholic acid	Reference
A. 1:1 mixture of ceric ammonium sulphate + molybdenum solution	brown	bluish black	brownish yellow	chocolate brown	[459]
B. 10% solution of molybdo-phosphoric acid in ethanol	greenish blue	bluish black	blue	blue	[240]
C. 5 g phosphomolybdic acid in 100 ml acetic acid + 5 ml concentrated sulphuric acid	dark blue	royal blue	dark blue	pale blue	[480]
D. 0.5 ml ansialdehyde in 1 ml concentrated sulphuric acid + 50 ml acetic acid	purple	blue	brown	bluish green	[241]
E. 20 g antimonytrichloride in 50 ml n-butanol mixed with 10 ml sulphuric acid + 20 ml acetic acid	yellowish green	greenish yellow	yellow	pinkish purple	[15]
F. 2 g ferric chloride in 83 ml n-butanol mixed with 15 ml concentrated sulphuric acid	greenish black	purplish black	brown	purplish black	[15]
G. Piece of copperwire dissolved in 0.5 g ammonium molybdate solution + 8.4 ml concentrated sulphuric acid + 80 ml distilled water	greenish yellow	purple	yellow	light purple	[169]

It should be emphasized that if the purified isotopes are to be stored for more than a few days or weeks before their administration, the purity should be reexamined as radiodecomposition may have occurred.

Labeling of Plasma Lipoproteins with Radioactive Cholesterol

All unesterified cholesterol present in plasma is in association with plasma lipoproteins; therefore, an ideal method for labeling plasma lipoproteins with radioactive cholesterol should ensure that the radioactive cholesterol is present in the same physiological state as the cholesterol native to the lipoproteins. The injection of radioactive precursors into intact animals is perhaps the most physiological method of labeling plasma cholesterol, but it also labels most other body pools of cholesterol simultaneously, which may or may not be undesirable. Feeding of radioactive cholesterol is another physiological method to label the liver-plasma pool of cholesterol; however, the absorption of radioactive cholesterol from the intestinal tract is rather slow and it also labels intestinal cholesterol which may or may not interfere with the planned study. Harvesting of plasma from donors a few hours after the injection of radioactive precursors is perhaps ideal in this regard, but the amounts of radioactive precursors necessary to yield high SA, plasma FC cannot be given to man with impunity.

Investigators have also taken aqueous suspensions of radioactive cholesterol in alcoholic saline and injected this unphysiological material i.v. for studies on the metabolism of plasma cholesterol [175, 215]. This indeed is the simplest method for labeling plasma lipoprotein cholesterol. Our studies indicated that the radioactive cholesterol injected in alcoholic saline having once been removed from circulation and reincorporated into plasma lipoproteins is metabolized in a fashion identical to that of cholesterol synthesized in the body or derived from the diet. This method, however, cannot be used for short-term studies where data during the first 24–48 h are required [431].

To overcome these drawbacks and to obtain a higher SA of plasma unesterified cholesterol, a number of in vitro methods have been proposed [18, 166, 357, 430, 496]; but for short-term studies on plasma cholesterol most of them have not been found satisfactory. The rate of clearance from circulation of radioactive cholesterol immediately after its i.v. injection depends on whether or not it is present in a physiological state. At least a part of the total unesterified cholesterol added to the plasma by most of the currently available methods did not appear to have the same characteristics as the cholesterol native to the lipoproteins, i.e. some of the tracer cholesterol appeared to leave the circulation at faster rates than the cholesterol present in the plasma [431].

In *Avigan*'s method, radioactive cholesterol is first adsorbed on an inert powder (celite) and it is then incubated with serum at 37 °C for 20 h in a mechanical shaker [18]. It has been shown that prolonged shaking at 37 °C denatures the plasma LDL [16], which was possibly responsible for the abnormally rapid rate of removal of the radioactive cholesterol incorporated into plasma from circulation by this method. Since incubation is carried out at 37 °C in the absence of a LCAT inhibitor, a considerable amount of radioactivity will also be associated with the plasma-esterified cholesterol.

The method of *Whereat and Staple* [496] utilizes Tween-20 to disperse the radioactive cholesterol in the serum. However, the presence of Tween-20 causes a marked increase in the rate of uptake of radioactive cholesterol and its subsequent catabolism by the liver [101].

In *Porte and Havel*'s method, radioactive cholesterol dissolved in ethanol is mixed with a 5% solution of albumin and then the ethanol is evaporated under an air stream. The albumin-stabilized cholesterol emulsion is then mixed with the serum to be labeled and allowed to stand for 1 h. Before using the plasma, the VLDL are removed [357]. It was shown by *Rose* [378] that the addition of ethanolic dispersion of cholesterol to serum results in the formation of particulate dispersions, the size of which depends on the concentration of cholesterol in the ethanolic solution. The radioactive cholesterol of large particles equilibrates slowly and to only a limited extent, while the radioactive cholesterol of small particles equilibrates with lipoprotein cholesterol at a reasonable rate.

Stokke and Norum [452] in their studies on esterification of plasma cholesterol found that albumin-stabilized emulsion prepared by dissolving cholesterol into ethanol was much less stable and gave less reproducible results in an LCAT assay system than that obtained by dissolving cholesterol in acetone. Another commonly used method is that of *Goodman and Noble* [166] which involves dissolving radioactive cholesterol in acetone and mixing the solution with plasma, incubating it at 37 °C for 2 h and then 16–20 h at room temperatures. This method is also subject to the same criticism.

A method of labeling plasma lipoproteins with radioactive cholesterol which utilized the physiological process of exchange of unesterified cholesterol between RBC and plasma was published in 1963 by *Sodhi and Kalant* [430]. This method involves the incubation of RBC in a solution of Tween-20

containing radioactive cholesterol. However, it was found that despite extensive washings of the labeled RBC, the Tween could not be removed from
the cells and therefore the original method was modified [434] in that albumin-stabilized solution instead of Tween-20 solution of radioactive cholesterol was used to label RBC. Also, RBC ghosts were used instead of fresh
RBC. Labeling of plasma with RBC ghosts is more convenient since the
ghosts can be stored for prolonged periods and thawed out as needed. This
appeared to be the better method than the others that it was compared with
[434] and it is therefore given in detail.

Preparation of RBC Ghosts

Fresh blood is collected from fasting normal donors in tubes containing
an anticoagulant. To obtain RBC, blood is centrifuged and the plasma and
the buffy coat are removed. RBC are then washed three times with physiological saline and suspended in the same solution. For hemolysis, the cells
are suspended in 10^{-4} EDTA. The pH is adjusted to 7.4 with tris (hydroxy-
methyl) aminomethane. The suspension is then centrifuged at 4°C for
15 min at 15,000 g. The supernatant is discarded and the pellet (ghosts) is
washed with the same solution (employed for hemolysis) with 0.017 M
sodium chloride added. Washings are carried out until the supernatant fluid
is free of hemoglobin color; this usually takes 5–7 washings. The final preparation of ghosts is then suspended in a suitable aliquot (usually 0.5–1 ml)
of physiological saline [340].

Preparation of Albumin-Stabilized Emulsion of Radioactive Cholesterol

The desired amount of purified radioactive cholesterol is evaporated to
dryness under a stream of nitrogen and dissolved in 0.5 ml of acetone. This
solution is then added slowly with continuous stirring to 5 ml of a 5% solution of human serum albumin in physiological saline. The solution is allowed
to stand for 20 min and then placed under a stream of nitrogen until the odor
of acetone is no longer detectable [357, 452].

Incorporation of Radioactive Cholesterol into RBC Ghosts

1 ml suspension of RBC ghosts is added to 5 ml of albumin-stabilized
emulsion of radioactive cholesterol in a 25- to 50-ml Erlenmeyer flask. The
mixture is then incubated at 37°C with gentle shaking for 16–20 h in a water
bath equipped with a mechanical shaker. At the end of the incubation period,
the ghosts are separated by centrifugation at 4°C and then washed twice
with at least 10 volumes of physiological saline to remove the albumin. They

are then resuspended in physiological saline. RBC ghosts may be dispensed in tubes in suitable aliquots, kept frozen ($-20\,°C$), and then thawed before use.

Incorporation of Radioactive Cholesterol into Plasma Lipoproteins

The radioactive ghosts are mixed with samples of fresh plasma to be labeled and incubated with gentle shaking at $4\,°C$ (to prevent esterification of plasma FC) for 16–20 h. The efficiency of the method is about 20%.

Labeling of plasma lipoproteins with radioactive cholesterol should be carried out under aseptic conditions. Before its injections, the plasma should be sterilized; this can be best accomplished by passing it through a millipore filter of 0.2 μm pore size.

Recently, *Akanuma et al.* [8] have described another method in a preliminary report for labeling plasma lipoproteins with radioactive cholesterol. The method involves coupling of plasma LDL to Sepharose activated with cyanogen bromide [205, 356]. The LDL-Sepharose complex is then incubated with radioactive cholesterol solution, which in turn is incubated with the plasma to be labeled. LDL-Sepharose is then removed from plasma before use.

Determination of SA of Cholesterol

If cholesterol is the only radioactive compound in the lipid mixture, it need not be isolated for determination of its SA. However if other lipids in the lipid mixture also contain the same isotope (^{14}C or ^{3}H) the radioactive cholesterol should be isolated by TLC (p. 15) or by precipitation with digitonin (p. 19). The lipid mixture or isolated cholesterol is dissolved in an organic solvent and two aliquots of known volume are taken out: one for the determination of the amount of cholesterol (p. 24–33) and the other for the determination of radioactivity (p. 117). The solvent is evaporated and the lipid(s) are picked up in the scintillation fluid for counting.

Chapter IV. Cholesterol Absorption

Cholesterol is relatively insoluble in water and is perhaps one of the largest molecules to be absorbed rather readily from the intestinal tract. Endogenous synthesis of cholesterol appears to be adequate for the normal growth and health of animals, and therefore it is not an essential ingredient of the human diet. Most of the cholesterol ingested by man comes from milk, animal fat, and eggs, and amounts to a total of 0.3–1.0 g per day. In normal subjects, the biliary cholesterol contributes additional 1.0–1.5 g; and in hypertriglyceridemic subjects the contributions from bile may be twice as much as those in normal subjects [432]. It is generally assumed that the exogenous and the endogenous cholesterol mix indistinguishably in the intestinal lumen and their absorption is therefore believed to be identical [55, 464, 465]. The amounts of cholesterol in intestinal secretions and in exfoliated cells are not considered important in man [115].

A number of successive steps can be delineated in the absorption of intestinal cholesterol: (1) transfer of FC to miceller phase; (2) transfer of FC from miceller phase into the mucosal cells; (3) esterification and incorporation of cholesterol into chylomicra and other intestinal lipoproteins and, finally, (4) transfer of FC and esterified cholesterol from mucosal cells into the lymph.

Most of the information on each of these steps is derived from studies on experimental animals, and it is only on the overall absorption of dietary cholesterol that some data are available for man. Although there are no reasons to believe that the formation of micelles, uptake of cholesterol by the intestinal mucosa, and its subsequent absorption are different in rat and man, there may well be significant differences in the overall absorption of cholesterol between man and experimental animals as suggested by the following:

In a rat, the lymphatic transport can be increased fivefold when a high cholesterol diet is given [466], and the SA of lymph cholesterol can be increased to about 90% of that of the dietary cholesterol [466]. Niether of these appear to occur in man. The addition of cholesterol to dietary fats does not increase the lymphatic transport of cholesterol in subjects with thoracic duct fistulae [60], and the maximum SA of lymph cholesterol attained in man is 25% of the SA of dietary cholesterol [60]. Despite these and other limitations [222], information available from experimental studies on absorption of cholesterol is generally relevant to man.

Most of the cholesterol entering the intestinal lumen is either already in the free form or is rapidly converted to FC by the pancreatic cholesterol esterase [463, 482]. Bile acids serve as cofactors for the activity of this enzyme [481], and in the presence of fatty acids and monoglycerides they also help in solubilization of cholesterol by forming miscelles [477].

The term 'absorption' implies that the cholesterol is not only picked up by the intestinal wall, but that it is also transported by the intestinal lymph into the circulation. The transfer of cholesterol from the intestinal lumen to the mucosa occurs by mass action [466, 467], but the absorption of cholesterol from the mucosal cells into the intestinal lymph is an active process involving incorporation of cholesterol into newly synthesized chylomicrons and lipoproteins. Experimental data suggest that the rate of cholesterol uptake by the intestinal mucosa can be much greater than the rate of its transfer out of the mucosa, so that when large amounts of cholesterol are fed to rats, there is a detectable increase in the cholesterol content of the intestinal wall [59]. In all likelihood, the rates of uptake into the mucosal cells of hydrolytic products of dietary triglycerides and of cholesterol are comparable, but it appears that the transfer out of the cell into the intestinal lymph is much faster for triglycerides and their products than for cholesterol. This difference in the rates of transfer from mucosal cells to the intestinal lymph between triglycerides and cholesterol and rapid turnover of intestinal cells may be critical in explaining why the absorption of dietary cholesterol is only half as efficient as the absorption of dietary triglycerides [48, 59, 464, 465].

Much of the absorption of dietary cholesterol and other fats occurs in the proximal small intestines since this is the first segment exposed to the bulk of dietary fats mixed with the bile. The mucosal cell lining the tips and upper halves of the villi incorporate more fats from the intestinal lumen than the cells near the bottoms of the villi or the cells lining the intestinal crypts [339]. Thus, the mucosal cells most active in the absorption of dietary fats have but the shortest time before they are exfoliated into the intestinal lumen during the normal process of their turnover. Thus, the overall rates of absorption of dietary fats may be determined by two independent processes, i.e. (a) the rates of their transfer out of cells into the lymph, and

(b) the life span of the mucosal cell containing the dietary lipids. The available information suggests that the rate of transport out of the cells into the lymph for triglycerides is so fast that little of their hydrolytic products taken up by the mucosal cells are lost in the exfoliated cells. In contrast, the rate of transfer of cholesterol from the intestinal wall into the lymph, relative to the turnover of mucosal cells, is slow enough that a significant proportion of the cholesterol taken up by the cells may still be contained in the cells when they are exfoliated into the intestinal lumen. Furthermore, the dietary cholesterol present in the exfoliated cells may not be as readily available for reabsorption as the cholesterol in the bile and diet, since cells may have to be disintegrated before the cellular cholesterol can be incorporated into micelles for absorption. When radioactive cholesterol was fed to rats, and the animals sacrificed at intervals the maximum radioactivity in the intestinal wall was present at the earliest time at which this determination was made, i.e. 1 h [56]. Thereafter, the radioactivity in the intestinal wall progressively declined, although there was still considerable radioactive cholesterol left in the intestinal lumen. These studies are in accord with the hypothesis that the cholesterol in the intestinal lumen in 1 h was not as readily available for absorption as the cholesterol initially fed to these rats.

Studies done on rats by *Wilson and Reinke* [502] indicated that about half of the cholesterol synthesized in the intestinal mucosa is secreted into the intestinal lumen, and only one half is absorbed into the intestinal lymph. They showed that there was little, if any, reabsorption of the cholesterol synthesized in the intestinal mucosa and then secreted into the lumen. Since the mucosal cells lining the tips of the villi synthesize cholesterol as actively as the cells in the crypts [277, 311, 427, 429], it is conceivable that the observations on synthesized cholesterol are comparable to those on the dietary cholesterol picked up by the mucosal cells. Work done in our laboratories is also in accord with the suggestion that a fraction of the dietary cholesterol taken up by the mucosal cells is returned to the intestinal lumen without ever entering the intestinal lymph [428].

It is well established that only FC can be taken up by the intestinal cells [158, 313, 462]. When intestinal mucosa is analyzed, most of the cholesterol present is also in the free form; and only a small fraction is present as CE. On the other hand, most of the cholesterol in the chylomicrons and the intestinal lipoproteins appearing in the intestinal lymph is esterified with long chain fatty acids [77, 46]. This suggests that the esterification of FC in the intestinal mucosa occurs just before the cholesterol is transported out of the intestines into the lymph. FC, phospholipids, and proteins, are present on the surface layer; whereas, the CE and triglycerides form the interior core of these particles [514, 521]. Studies in rabbits suggested that under certain conditions, intestinal VLDL may transport more cholesterol than chylomicrons [368, 388, 525]. It is not yet clear how important are the intestinal VLDL for the transport of dietary cholesterol in man.

Our studies in rats suggested that the fractional rate of transport from intestinal mucosa to the intestinal lymph was about three times greater for dietary cholesterol than for the cholesterol synthesized in the intestinal cells [437].

Unabsorbed cholesterol is acted upon by the microorganisms in the large gut and is converted to a number of other steroids before its excretion in the feces. In germ-free rats, all of the unabsorbed cholesterol appears as cholesterol in the feces [99]. The predominant fecal metabolite of unabsorbed cholesterol in man is coprostanol; and small amounts of coprostanone and unchanged cholesterol are also seen [381, 426]. It is necessary, therefore, to determine each of these derivatives of cholesterol quantitatively to estimate the total quantities of cholesterol lost in the feces.

Normal diet also contains considerable amounts of plant sterols. The major component of dietary plant sterols is β-sitosterol; others, such as campesterol, stigmasterol, and brassicasterol are also found in small amounts. Given in large doses, plant sterols can inhibit the absorption of dietary cholesterol [180, 201], but the amounts generally present in ordinary diets do not have such an effect. As against approximately 40% absorption of cholesterol [57, 249, 361, 362], the absorption of β-sitosterol is less than 5% [170, 390]. Campesterol is absorbed a little better than β-sitosterol [253]. An inherited disorder leading to the increased absorption of dietary β-sitosterol has recently been described in 2 sisters with extensive tendon xanthomas and normal cholesterol levels [35].

The unabsorbed β-sitosterol is also acted upon by intestinal microorganisms in the same manner as the unabsorbed cholesterol [179, 247, 248].

Grundy et al. [179] presented evidence suggesting that there were considerable losses of dietary cholesterol and β-sitosterol despite careful and meticulous methodology employed for their recoveries in the feces. They postulated that the losses (or incomplete recovery) of these sterols were due to the degradation of the sterol nucleus. They also presented evidence suggesting that the percent degradation of unabsorbed cholesterol in the intestinal lumen was identical to the percent degradation of dietary β-sitosterol. It was suggested that the losses of cholesterol should be monitored by determining the fecal recoveries of dietary β-sitosterol in all studies on cholesterol absorption [179]. These 'unaccounted for' losses are seen mainly in subjects consuming liquid formula diets [110], and not in subjects consuming natural solid food diets [110, 237, 247, 248].

Methods to Study Absorption of Dietary Cholesterol

A number of different methods are available for determining the absorption of dietary cholesterol in man. It is important that the pros and cons of all available methods are considered before choosing the appropriate method for the study. All the methods involve the use of radioactive cholesterol which is administered either i.v. or orally or both. Simultaneous feeding of radioactive β-sitosterol is also involved in some methods, while feeding of markers such as chromic oxide and carmine red are necessary in others. The various methods may be subdivided into two broad groups. One group is characterized by measurements during metabolic steady-state conditions so that the results reflect the net absorption of dietary cholesterol over a 24-hour period. These methods are not meant to show whether or not there are any differences in the absorption at different times of the day or from different meals. These methods also exclude the possibility of errors due to isotopic exchange between the cholesterol in the intestinal lumen and in the intestinal wall. The second group of methods involves determinations after a single administration of radioactive cholesterol and as such are subject to possible errors due to the isotopic exchange, but they allow quick comparison of percentage absorption of cholesterol in different metabolic conditions. On cholesterol-free diets these procedures permit measurement of the absorption of recirculated cholesterol of endogenous origin. Most of these methods are based on estimations of the differences between dietary intake and the recovery of unabsorbed dietary neutral steroids in feces, and they differ according to the way in which the amounts of unabsorbed dietary sterol is calculated.

Methods for the Measurement of Dietary Cholesterol Absorption during Steady-State Conditions

Method 1
This method involves the combined use of isotopic and chromatographic sterol balance methods, and was developed by *Grundy and Ahrens* [175]. The

details of this method are given on page 118. The values for absorbed dietary cholesterol are obtained as follows:

Dietary cholesterol absorbed (mg/day) = cholesterol intake (mg/day) – unabsorbed dietary cholesterol (mg/day), where,

Unabsorbed dietary cholesterol (mg/day) = fecal total neutral steroids (mg/day) – fecal endogenous neutral steroids (mg/day).

In this method, the fecal total neutral steroids are determined by the combined use of a TLC and GLC methods (chromatographic balance, page 127), and the fecal endogenous neutral steroids are estimated isotopically (isotopic balance, p. 127). Both fecal total and endogenous neutral steroids should be corrected for losses and for variations in fecal flow as explained in the next section.

Method 2

The only difference between this and the method 1 is the way in which the amounts of fecal total neutral steroids are estimated. In this method, both the fecal total and endogenous neutral steroids are estimated by the isotopic balance method [199, 509]. This method is based on the assumption that in the absence of dietary cholesterol the SA of excreted neutral steroids is essentially the same as that of plasma cholesterol. This is reasonable since the two sources of fecal neutral steroids are bile cholesterol and cholesterol of the intestinal mucosa, both of which are in isotopic equilibrium with plasma cholesterol. In the steady state, when cholesterol is being ingested, the extent by which the SA of fecal cholesterol is lower than that of plasma cholesterol reflects the dilution of excreted endogenous cholesterol with unabsorbed dietary cholesterol. Fecal total neutral steroids by this method are calculated as follows:

Fecal total neutral steroids (mg/day) = total radioactivity in neutral steroids fraction (dpm/day) ÷ SA of the *fecal* cholesterol (dpm/mg).

Absorption of dietary cholesterol is then calculated as described above in method 1.

The total fecal neutral steroids (estimated from the total radioactivity in the neutral steroid fractions and the SA of fecal cholesterol) would include all the unabsorbed cholesterol whether of dietary or of endogenous origin. These estimates should be similar to those determined by methods involving TLC and GLC. *Grundy and Ahrens* [175] examined this in 1 subject and we examined the same in 10 of our subjects. We examined a total of 100, 3-day fecal pools obtained before and during treatment with clofibrate and nicotinic acid. The dietary cholesterol intake in these subjects ranged from 401 to 1,214 mg per day. Fecal total neutral steroids were determined both by chromatographic methods (TLC and GLC) and isotopic methods (from SA of fecal coprostanol) and the total radioactivity in neutral steroid fractions of the fecal extracts. The values obtained by isotopic methods were $5\pm10\%$ lower than those given by the chromatographic methods (table II). The correlation between the two methods was excellent ($r = 0.92$). Although the treatment with clofibrate or nicotinic acid caused increases in the excretion of fecal neutral steroids in some of the subjects, estimates obtained by the two methods remained comparable as they were before the treatments [246].

In the chromatographic method, corrections for the fecal recovery of dietary β-sitosterol does not take into account the absorption of β-sitosterol. The corrections are made for 100% recovery of β-sitosterol in the feces as if none of the dietary β-sitosterol is absorbed from the intestinal tract. However, β-sitosterol is absorbed up to about 5% so that the corrections should have been made, not for 100% of its recovery, but somewhere between 95 and 100%, which would bring the values obtained by chromatographic methods much closer to those obtained by the radioisotopic method. It would appear then that even in studies where the diets contain cholesterol, the use of isotopic methods give reliable estimates of the total fecal neutral steroids. In the 1 subject where the two methods were compared, there was less than 2% difference between the two methods [175].

For calculations of fecal total neutral steroids, the SA of fecal cholesterol could be substituted by the SA of coprostanol or coprostanone, the two major bacterial metabolites of cholesterol in feces. The SA of fecal cholesterol is generally lower than the SA of coprostanol, although it has a slightly lower SA than that of coprostanone. The differences, however, were only $1.5\pm1.2\%$. Since coprostanol is by far the largest neutral steroid present in the feces (65–90%), it would appear to be the most appropriate compound for the determination of the SA of fecal neutral steroids.

The SA of fecal cholesterol or coprostanol can be determined by preliminary isolation of major fecal neutral steroid bands by TLC on silica gel G using ether:heptane (45:55 v/v). Radioactivity is then determined in one aliquot and the mass by GLC in another (p. 129). In laboratories where GLC facilities are not available, the plant sterols could be separated from cholesterol by the reverse-phase TLC (described in detail, p. 22) [111], and the cholesterol can be estimated colorimetrically or enzymatically (p. 25, 30). The advantage of this method is that only one band needs to be analyzed instead

Table II. Comparison of values of fecal neutral steroids determined by GLC and by isotopic balance method

Subject No.	Number of 3-day pools	Before treatment			Number of 3-day pools	During treatment		
		GLC mg/day	isotopic mg/day	difference %		GLC mg/day	isotopic mg/day	difference %
1	5	918±186	800±128	12±7	7	971±107	862±91	11±6
2	4	1,276±145	1,100±90	13±9	6	1,219±44	1,084±83	11±4
3	5	1,283±74	1,160±87	9±6	6	1,296±158	1,200±162	7±8
4	3	407±9	356±31	12±6	5	603±34	559±41	7±3
5	6	717±91	652±89	9±5	5	916±82	825±88	10±5
5a	–	–	–	–	4	864±49	818±46	5±5
6	3	682±200	635±207	8±5	4	1,097±108	1,057±108	4±2
7	3	1,113±157	1,021±175	9±3	5	1,100±70	1,060±87	7±3
8	4	788±60	899±77	-14±6	4	1,004±43	1,142±115	-14±6
9	4	1,100±58	1,210±103	-10±6	4	1,387±407	1,513±444	-10±10
10	3	816±84	826±68	-1±3	5	759±17	813±14	-7±3
10a	–	–	–	–	5	772±109	820±132	-6±5
Mean ± SD				5±10				3±10
Correlation(r)				0.92				0.91

of three, thus saving a considerable amount of time. Secondly, the absorption of cholesterol can be estimated in laboratories where GLC facilities are not available.

Both of these methods share common advantages and disadvantages. The absorption of dietary cholesterol can be measured daily by any of these methods. Both methods require i.v. administration of at least 25 μCi of radioactive cholesterol, making it unsuitable in subjects in whom use of the radioactivity is not advisable. Although the calculations can be made both immediately and repeatedly, reliable calculations can be made only after the SA-time curve becomes log-linear, which usually takes anywhere between 3 and 6 weeks.

The transit time of the intestinal contents must either be measured (by feeding markers such as carmine red) or simply assumed. The calculations of endogenous neutral steroids depend on knowing the plasma cholesterol SA at the time when labeled biliary cholesterol is secreted into the intestinal lumen. When the SA-time curve is falling rapidly or if the turnover of intestinal contents is sluggish, or both, the results will have diminished validity. The following other discrepancies can also occur. If cholesterol synthesized in liver or intestinal mucosa is excreted into the intestinal lumen before it reaches isotopic equilibrium with plasma cholesterol, e.g. under conditions such as cholestyramine treatment and surgical bypass of the terminal ileum, the radioactivity of fecal sterols will be diluted to some undefined degree [176, 181]. In a similar fashion, the sterols ingested by animals licking their fur dilutes the radioactivity of the fecal neutral steroids.

Our results suggest that the isotopic method is *nearly* as good as the chromatographic method for estimating fecal steroids. If the amount of cholesterol in the diet is known, the amount absorbed can be determined by an isotopic balance method without the use of GLC. The latter is essential if the estimates of intestinal degradation of neutral steroids are required. If a chromatographic method is not available, the same information can be obtained by feeding a subject a known dose of radioactive β-sitosterol and calculating its recovery in the fecal pools, collected over the next 8 days. Generally, the degradation of dietary and endogenous cholesterol does not appear to be an important factor in most subjects given solid food diets [247, 248].

Method 3

This method is based on the isotopic steady-state concept developed by *Morris et al.* [307]. The method involves feeding radioactive cholesterol of a known SA until the plasma cholesterol SA reaches a plateau. *Morris et al.* [307] did not make any quantitative estimates for the cholesterol absorbed or synthesized but estimated only the relative contributions of dietary and newly synthesized cholesterol to the plasma pool by comparing the SA of cholesterol of plasma (after it reaches the plateau) to the SA of dietary cholesterol. Use of this method for the quantitative estimation of absorbed cholesterol was suggested by *Grundy and Ahrens* [176]. With this method, absorbed cholesterol can be estimated anytime after 4 days of continuous isotope feeding and without the necessity of obtaining an isotopic steady state [176]. The radioactive cholesterol used in oral labeling should be incorporated in the diet and fed in different meals during the day to ensure continuous intake of radioactive cholesterol.

$$Z = X + Y,$$

where Z = total fecal neutral steroids (mg/day), X = fecal neutral steroids of endogenous origin (mg/day), Y = unabsorbed dietary cholesterol (mg/day), and

$$Z.SA_{(Z)} = X.SA_{(X)} + Y.SA_{(Y)}$$

where $SA_{(Z)}$, $SA_{(X)}$ and $SA_{(Y)}$ represent the SA of fecal total neutral steroids, plasma cholesterol and dietary cholesterol, respectively. After solving for Y, the absorbed cholesterol is calculated as the difference between dietary intake and unabsorbed dietary cholesterol (Y).

Method 4

This method was proposed by *Wilson and Lindsey* [501] in 1965 and is a modification of the isotopic steady-state method described above. By this method, absorption of dietary cholesterol is calculated as follows:

Dietary cholesterol absorbed (mg/day) = daily cholesterol turnover (mg/day) × fraction of plasma cholesterol derived from the absorbed cholesterol

Cholesterol in plasma derived from absorbed cholesterol (%) = plasma cholesterol SA (dpm/mg) × 100 ÷ dietary cholesterol SA (dpm/mg).

Daily cholesterol turnover can be estimated by either the sterol balance method or isotope kinetic method (p. 64, 68). This method is valid only in isotopic steady-state conditions; the criteria for which are: (1) an unchanging level of SA of plasma cholesterol, and (2) the amount of radioactive cholesterol fed each day is matched by the amounts excreted in the feces.

Methods 3 and 4 are both sound theoretically. However, if calculations for absorption of dietary cholesterol are made by method 4 prior to the attainment of isotopic steady state, the calculated values would be erroneously low. The major disadvantage of method 4 is the exceedingly long period required for the SA of plasma cholesterol to reach a plateau. This period could be shortened by giving a large priming dose of radioactivity at the beginning of the study, either orally or i.v. [176].

In a comparative study, *Quintao et al.* [361, 362] found method 3 to be superior to the others in precision and reproducibility. The main advantage is that the unabsorbed dietary cholesterol is calculated directly and with great precision because the major proportion of the excreted radioactivity is in that fraction. Furthermore, corrections need not be made for undefined lags in transit of intestinal contents. However, constant feeding of daily doses of radioactive cholesterol for three or four stool collections requires a minimum of 2 weeks. These methods (3 and 4) cannot be used for the estimation of dietary cholesterol absorption in conditions where there is any appreciable contribution of nonlabeled cholesterol to the intestinal lumen from sources other than from the diet [176, 361, 362].

Methods for Measurement of Dietary Cholesterol Absorption during Nonsteady-State Conditions

Method 5
This method was proposed by *Borgström* [57]. It involves simultaneous oral administration of a test dose containing radioactive cholesterol and radioactive β-sitosterol. (Labels used should be different, e.g. ^{14}C-cholesterol and ^{3}H β-sitosterol or vice versa.) Feces are then collected for a period of 8 days and pooled. Fecal neutral steroids are then extracted from an aliquot and the radioactivity measured. The absorption of dietary cholesterol is calculated as percentage of the administered dose not recovered in the feces.

Percentage of dietary cholesterol absorbed = (1-[radioactivity in fecal cholesterol ÷ radioactivity in fecal β-sitosterol] × [radioactivity in fed β-sitosterol ÷ radioactivity in fed cholesterol]) × 100.

Use of β-sitosterol circumvents the problem of losses due to degradation or other reasons.

This is a relatively simple and rapid method. It requires only small amounts of radioactivity: as low as 0.5–1 μCi of each sterol. Absorption can be measured frequently and under any experimental conditions. When the diet is free of cholesterol, this method permits the measurement of the absorption of recirculated cholesterol of endogenous origin. The major drawback of this method is the collection of feces for 8 consecutive days, during which time some of the cholesterol having once been absorbed may also be lost in the feces through its excretion in the bile. However, the errors introduced by this method are very small.

Method 6 (Fecal Ratio Method)

In 1971, we proposed another method for estimating absorbed dietary cholesterol in man. This method involves feeding a mixture of ^{3}H-cholesterol and ^{14}C-β-sitosterol (in a known ratio) and $\simeq$ 300 mg of carmine red. A fecal specimen containing *maximum red color* is obtained and extracted for neutral steroids. The ratio of the two isotopes is determined and the percentage of the dietary cholesterol absorbed is calculated from the equation:

$$\frac{X - Y}{X} \times 100.$$

X is the ratio of the two radiosterols in the administered dose and Y is the ratio in the 'test' fecal specimen. It is not necessary to obtain complete stool collections or to quantitate the two radioactive sterols as long as the ratios of the two isotopes in the administered material and in the fecal specimen are known. It is, however, important to analyze the fecal specimen containing *maximum red color*, which is not necessarily the first sample of feces collected. This is the sample which contains most of the unabsorbed radiosterols [435].

This method has been validated in rats and in man [438]. It was shown by *Quintao et al.* [361, 362] that the results obtained by *Borgström*'s method (method 5) are nearly the same as those obtained by other more reliable methods (methods 1 and 3). Our studies indicate that the results obtained by the 'fecal ratio method' are on average 2% higher than those obtained by *Borgström*'s method, and the correlation between the two methods is also excellent (r = 0.89).

The critical proof for the validity of our method (at least in rats) was given by the actual determinations of total radioactivity in the carcasses of animals given the isotopes by gastric intubation. The percentage absorption calculated by the ratio method was in remarkable agreement with values determined by the carcass analysis. The correlation between the two methods was excellent (r = 0.95) [438].

The use of β-sitosterol as a marker for cholesterol absorption circumvents the need for determination of degradation or any other losses of cholesterol in the intestinal tract. The determination of the ratio in a single specimen of feces is considerably simpler than determining the total amounts of radioactivity in the 8-day fecal pools. This method can be used in out-patients and also to compare the effects of diets or drugs on cholesterol absorption.

One drawback of this method is that the absorption of cholesterol can-not be measured by estimating the ratio of radiosterols in any fecal sample collected casually after feeding the two radiosterols. *The calculations are valid only if the ratio is estimated from the fecal specimens containing the bulk of unabsorbed dietary sterols.*

When radioactive cholesterol and β-sitosterol are given by a single oral dose, the ratios of the two isotopes show progressive changes with each successive passage of feces. *Quintao et al.* [361, 362], believed that the low ratio of the isotopes in the first fecal specimen reflected the disappearance of the labeled cholesterol into the intestinal mucosa by *isotopic exchange*, and the subsequent increasing ratios suggested to them that there was a back exchange of this labeled cholesterol in the mucosa with the cholesterol in the intestinal lumen. Experimental work done in rats did indeed suggest that some of the cholesterol incorporated into the intestinal mucosa is secreted back into the intestinal lumen [438]. However, it is not yet clear whether this occurs as a result of isotopic exchange between the cholesterol in the lumen and that in the intestinal mucosa, or if it occurs through ex-foliation of mucosal cells into the intestinal lumen. In man, the increase seen in the ratios of the two isotopes in successive fecal samples may also have been due to the resecretion of absorbed radioactive cholesterol through the biliary tract. Whatever the reasons for the increasing ratios, the bulk of the unabsorbed radioactive sterols are excreted in feces rather rapidly (36–72 h), and only small fractions are seen in later samples.

Patients with aβ-lipoproteinemia can incorporate cholesterol into the mucosal cells, but it is held there since it cannot be transported out into the intestinal lymph. For these specific reasons, the absorption cannot be calcu-lated from the ratios of the two isotopes in the sample of feces containing most of the unabsorbed dietary sterols in such patients.

A modification of this method was recently suggested by *Crouse* [93].

Method 7 (Plasma Ratio Method)

A dual isotope 'plasma ratio method' for measurement of cholesterol absorption was proposed by *Zilversmit* [523]. The method depends on oral administration of cholesterol labeled with an isotope and i.v. administration of colloidal suspension of cholesterol labeled with another isotope. The percent absorption of cholesterol is calculated as follows:

$$\frac{\text{Percent of oral dose in an aliquot of plasma}}{\text{Percentage of i.v. dose in the same aliquot of plasma}} \times 100.$$

The ratio is measured 48 h or longer after the administration of the isotopes.

This method is based on the assumption that the absorbed portion of an orally administered dose is distributed and metabolized in the same manner as an i.v. administered dose. It has been shown in other studies [335, 431] that labeled colloidal cholesterol is quickly removed from plasma after its i.v. injection and then gradually released into the blood stream so that over a 4-day period the SA-time curve corresponded in shape to that generated by an oral dose of cholesterol. The cholesterol for i.v. administration should not be solubilized in Tween-20.

Zilversmit and Hughes [524] have validated the method in rats. They have shown that the values for cholesterol absorption under different conditions, obtained by a dual isotope plasma ratio method, are similar to the values obtained by fecal analysis of orally administered isotope according to *Borgström's* method. *Samuel et al.* [394] compared the plasma ratio method with *Borgström's* method in man on a cholesterol intake of 75–760 mg/day. They found that the plasma ratio remained constant after 72 h. The difference between the two methods was $\pm 7\%$.

This is a simple method and is not dependent on fecal collections, and as such is independent of possible sterol degradation in the intestinal tract. One blood sample taken at any time after 4 days of isotope administration will suffice and the test can be repeated. Because of its simplicity, the dual isotope plasma ratio method is suitable for screening a large outpatient population.

Chapter V. Cholesterol Synthesis

It is now well recognized that almost every animal tissue is capable of at least some degree of cholesterol synthesis [115]. An outline of the pathway for cholesterol synthesis from acetate is given in figure 5. The first step is the activation of acetate by the coenzyme A, and then two molecules of acetyl-CoA are catalyzed to form acetoacetyl-CoA by an enzyme called β-ketothiolase [197, 227]. Acetoacetyl-CoA serves as an intermediate for synthesis of fatty acids, ketone bodies, as well as cholesterol [271]. Acetoacetyl-CoA condenses with another molecule of acetyl-CoA to form β-hydroxy-β-methylglutaryl-CoA (HMG-CoA) [363, 389]. The latter compound can either be converted to ketone bodies or to cholesterol [272]. The conversion of HMG-CoA to mevalonic acid by HMG-CoA reductase is the irreversible step in cholesterol biosynthesis, and it is generally believed that most, if not all, of mevalonate is incorporated into cholesterol [43, 472].

Mevalonate is converted through a series of steps to form farnesyl pyrophosphate and squalene. Squalene is an open-chain hydrocarbon which upon cyclization is converted to lanosterol. The lanosterol could be converted to cholesterol either via desmosterol (unsaturated side chain series) or via Δ7-cholestenol (saturated side chain series) as shown in figure 7. Details of the cholesterol synthetic pathway can be found in excellent reviews recently published [43, 109, 239].

The rates of cholesterol synthesis differ markedly from one tissue to another. Experimental data on rats [113] and monkeys [114] indicate that the highest rates of cholesterol synthesis per unit weight of tissue occurs in liver and in the ileum. Of the total cholesterol synthesized in the body, more than 80% is produced in the liver, about 10% in the gastrointestinal tract, and about 5% by the skin; the remainder is synthesized in all other tissues together. These figures are derived from experimental animals, and it is generally believed that they also reflect the state in man. In accord with these observations in experimental animals, biopsy specimens demonstrated that the synthesis of cholesterol in human liver was more active than in any other human tissue examined [115]. Biopsy specimens from the gastrointes-

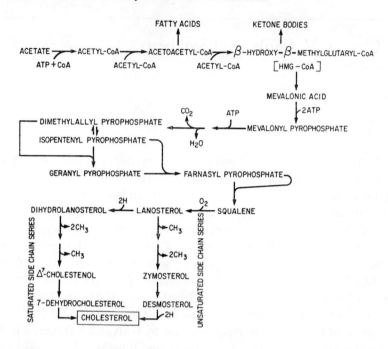

Fig. 7. An outline of the pathway for the biosynthesis of cholesterol.

tinal tract of man also showed that the pattern of synthesis in the intestinal tract in man was similar to that observed in experimental animals [116].

The available evidence from studies in rats indicate that there is a circadian rhythm in biosynthesis of cholesterol both in liver and in intestines [22, 126, 231]. Cholesterol synthesis gradually increases through the day reaching a maximum between 8 p.m. and midnight, and decreases again to a minimum at approximately 8 a.m. [191, 404]. Comparable information for man is not available.

Considerable attention has recently been focused on cholesterol synthesis in fibroblasts, smooth muscle cells, and leukocytes to delineate metabolic defects in familial hypercholesterolemia [37, 69, 144]. These studies have yielded important information on the catabolism of plasma lipoproteins and on the mechanisms of control of cholesterol synthesis in these tissues when cultured and incubated *in vitro*. However, it is important to bear in mind that the fraction of total cholesterol synthesized in the body by these peripheral tissues is rather small. Furthermore, these tissues do not synthesize lipoproteins, and the mechanisms of their contributions to plasma choles-terol, if any, are not known.

It was shown by *Taylor and Gould* [473] and *Gould et al.* [172], and sub sequently by many others, that the ability to synthesize cholesterol by the liver slices from animals fed high cholesterol diets is markedly reduced if radioactive acetate is used as a precursor. However, if radioactive mevalonate is used, marked inhibition as seen with radioactive acetate was not observed [171]. This negative feedback control of cholesterol synthesis from acetate has been shown to operate at the level of HMG-CoA reductase which con-verts HMG-CoA to mevalonate [416]. Studies carried out with liver, intes-tines, skin fibroblasts, smooth muscle cells, and leukocytes and a number of other tissues all demonstrate that the control of cholesterol synthesis is at the same level [14, 69, 415]. The implication is that a greater fraction of the precursor acetate pool enters the pathway for cholesterol synthesis in condi-tions of increased cholesterol synthesis. Similarly, a smaller proportion of available acetate precursor pool enters the cholesterol pathway when choles-terol synthesis is decreased. A number of other metabolic pathways are available for its metabolism, and only a small fraction of the available acetate pool enters the cholesterol pathway.

It appears that there are at least two intracellular pools of acetyl-CoA; one is intramitochondrial generated within the mitochondria from oxidation of endogenous substrates such as fatty acids, and the other is extramitochon-drial. The two pools are not in rapid equilibrium with each other because the penetration of acetate into mitochondria is rather slow. The synthesis of cholesterol occurs predominantly from extramitochondrial acetate, whereas the synthesis of ketones or production of carbon dioxide occurs from the intramitochondrial acetyl-CoA [87, 88, 369, 457].

It is generally believed that once the acetate is converted into mevalonate for all practical purposes it has no other pathway but to be incorporated into cholesterol sooner or later. If this indeed is true, changes in the synthetic rates of cholesterol will not significantly influence the *proportion* of the mevalonate *ultimately* incorporated into cholesterol, although the time taken for the complete incorporation may be affected. Therefore, the i.v. injection of mevalonate may be used as a standard for determining the changes in the proportion of acetate incorporated into cholesterol in different experimental conditions. This concept, however, is not supported by the recent work from Dr. *Ahren*'s laboratories [269, 288].

Liver is the most important organ for cholesterol synthesis in the body, and cholesterol synthesized by the liver has a number of available pathways.

They are: (1) incorporation into cellular and subcellular membranes in the structure of the liver; (2) incorporation into plasma lipoproteins and secretion into circulation; (3) conversion of cholesterol into bile acids and their secretion in the bile; (4) secretion of cholesterol as such in the bile, and (5) storage as CE.

Preliminary data from investigations of *Bricker et al.* [66] and from our own laboratories [429, 439, 440] indicate that most of the recently synthesized cholesterol in the liver appears in plasma lipoproteins and the amounts excreted directly in the bile either as cholesterol or as newly synthesized bile acids are relatively small. It is also conceivable that an appreciable fraction of plasma LDL is catabolized in the peripheral tissues, thus necessitating transfer of large amounts of cholesterol in plasma from tissues back into liver.

Within minutes after its i.v. injection, the radioactive cholesterol distributes itself in the plasma compartment and the subsequent isotopic exchange between plasma and tissues results in distribution of the injected radioactivity in the total exchangeable cholesterol pool. This isotopic exchange by definition precludes any net transfer or turnover. Turnover involves the entry of net amounts of unlabeled cholesterol and the exit of equal fractions of labeled and unlabeled cholesterol from exchangeable pools under steady-state conditions. The cholesterol entering the exchangeable pools comes either from *de novo* synthesis or from absorption of dietary cholesterol. The exit of cholesterol from the exchangeable pools occurs in the form of biliary cholesterol and newly synthesized bile acids which are ultimately lost in the feces.

When a lipoprotein labeled with radioactive cholesterol is mixed with another labeled lipoprotein, there is a rapid isotopic exchange of FC present in the two lipoproteins, so that by the time the liporpoteins are reisolated (by preparative ultracentrifugation), the SA of the FC in both classes of lipoproteins becomes almost equal. Similarly, when plasma labeled with radioactive cholesterol is mixed with unlabeled RBC and the mixture is allowed to incubate at 37 °C, the SA of FC in RBC begins to increase and in about 4 h the SA of FC in plasma and in RBC becomes equal [124, 187, 430]. When radioactive precursors of cholesterol are injected i.v., the SA of liver cholesterol goes up rapidly, and the SA of plasma cholesterol also becomes equal to that of liver FC within 2–4 h [82, 173]. This has been interpreted to mean that the rates of isotopic exchange between the liver FC and plasma FC are very rapid. However, it is necessary to keep in mind that the equilibration of SA of liver FC and plasma FC in the latter instance is brought about by the secretion of radioactive cholesterol by the liver into plasma lipoproteins, as well as by the phenomenon of isotopic exchange. Conversely, there is a rapid transfer of radioactive cholesterol from plasma into liver when plasma is pulse-labeled with radioactive cholesterol (in a physiological state). A part of this equilibration also is due to the net transfer of plasma cholesterol into the liver. It is therefore worth emphasizing that the isotopic exchange is not necessarily the only mechanism by which equilibration of SA between cholesterol pools occurs.

Depending on the rates of equilibration of SA between plasma and tissue cholesterol pools, the tissue cholesterol is designated either as readily exchangeable or slowly exchangeable. True to precursor-product relationships, the differences between the SA values of tissue and plasma cholesterol pools at or after equilibration depend on the rates of exchange and the relative sizes of the tissue cholesterol pools. The slower the rate of exchange and the larger the relative size of the product pool, the greater will be the difference in SA of cholesterol in the two compartments [521].

Within minutes after its i.v. injection, radioactive cholesterol distributes itself in the plasma compartment, and its further rate of decay is given by a slope which can be broken into 2 or 3 exponentials depending upon the period of observation [166, 167, 392]. The terminal exponential portion of the slope is dependent on the turnover of total exchangeable cholesterol in the body. The slope is determined by the amounts of unlabeled cholesterol entering the system from either *de novo* synthesis or from absorption of dietary cholesterol. To a minor degree, the slope is also influenced, in the reverse direction, by the isotopic exchange of cholesterol between plasma and tissue pools. By the time the decline in the SA of plasma FC becomes exponential, different exchangeable pools must have reached equilibrium with the SA of plasma cholesterol. Since the tissue cholesterol pools tend to have higher SA than the plasma FC, the continuous isotopic exchange between tissue and plasma FC pools would tend to decrease the slope of decay. Analysis of the SA slope of plasma FC can provide estimates for the turnover of cholesterol and other parameters of cholesterol metabolism [166, 328, 392]. It is worth nothing that the values of cholesterol turnover derived from the data on plasma cholesterol SA refer to total cholesterol in exchangeable pools and not to plasma compartment alone. As described in the next section, the turnover of plasma cholesterol is defined as the net amount of cholesterol entering and leaving plasma per unit time, whereas, the 'turnover of endogenous cholesterol' includes the total cholesterol derived from endogenous synthesis and from absorption of the dietary cholesterol. On a cholesterol-free diet, therefore, the turnover equals cholesterol synthesis.

Turnover of Plasma Cholesterol

There is neither synthesis nor degradation of cholesterol in plasma. Therefore, the cholesterol has to come from tissues into plasma, and for its degradation it has to go back from plasma into the tissues. By definition, the turnover implies the net amount of cholesterol which enters plasma per unit time and in steady-state conditions, it equals the amount of cholesterol leaving plasma to go into tissues. Isotopic exchange of FC between plasma and tissues is by definition precluded from the considerations of *metabolic* turnover.

The entry of cholesterol into plasma from the intestines is in the form of large molecules called chylomicra or other lipoproteins synthesized in the intestines. The contributions to plasma cholesterol by liver are in the form of either VLDL, possibly of some of the LDL, and the HDL. Tissues other than the intestines and liver do not synthesize lipoproteins; therefore, any contributions from such tissues is in the form or forms which are not yet understood. However, all cholesterol in plasma is transported in association with specific proteins and other lipids of plasma lipoproteins. After a fatty meal containing cholesterol, the intestinal mucosa incorporates the dietary as well as biliary cholesterol into chylomicra and other lipoproteins which are then delivered to plasma through the intestinal lymph. The rates of its entry into and clearance from plasma are such that even during the absorption of a meal loaded with cholesterol, the increases in plasma levels of this lipid are relatively minor. It has been shown in rats that most of the chyle cholesterol entering the circulation is rapidly removed by the liver [163, 327, 367], although under certain conditions small but significant fractions may also be removed by extrahepatic tissues [270, 402]. During absorption, therefore, the term 'turnover of plasma cholesterol' will also include the cholesterol entering the circulation in the form of chylomicra (and other intestinal lipoproteins). During the postabsorptive phase, however, liver constitutes the most important source of plasma cholesterol. The liver synthesizes VLDL, HDL (and possibly undetermined amounts of LDL). Also, small but significant amounts of cholesterol may enter plasma from the extrahepatic tissues. Therefore, one should estimate the contributions of cholesterol entering plasma in chyle, from liver, and from extrahepatic tissues. Since the fluctuations in the levels of plasma cholesterol are not marked, the amounts of cholesterol which leave plasma almost equal the amounts entering plasma.

Although there is some information about the modes of cholesterol entering plasma, little information is available as to how it leaves plasma.

It is known that the cholesterol from chylomicra and VLDL [133, 163] enters the liver. Recent studies have also shown that a fraction of the circulating plasma LDL can be bound and degraded by the peripheral tissues [69, 70, 448, 449]. It is obvious that most of the cholesterol released from the catabolism of plasma lipoproteins will have to be transported to the liver for its ultimate catabolism and elimination. Because of this, any cholesterol which is released by the lipoproteins in the peripheral tissues will have to reenter the circulation in association with some plasma lipoproteins for its transport back to the liver. In summary, the term 'turnover of plama cholesterol' includes considerations of transport of cholesterol from plasma to the tissues and from the tissues to plasma.

Methods to Study Cholesterol Synthesis in Man

A number of different methods are available for the estimation of cholesterol synthesis in man. Most of the methods involve the use of radioisotopes of cholesterol or its precursors such as acetate and mevalonate. The methods available can generally be divided as follows:

(A) Quantitative methods. (a) Sterol balance methods: (1) isotope balance, (2) chromatographic balance, and (3) combined isotope and chromatographic balance. (b) Kinetic analysis of plasma cholesterol SA curves based on: (1) two-pool model, (2) three-pool model, and (3) input-output analysis. (c) Isotope steady-state methods. (d) Methods for nonsteady-state conditions.

(B) Qualitative methods, (a) Relative rates of acetate and mevalonate incorporation into plasma FC. (b) Determination of squalene and methyl sterols in plasma. (c) Determination of hepatic-3-hydroxy-3-methylglutaryl-CoA reductase activity.

Quantitative Methods

These methods give absolute values for the total body synthesis, and they require metabolic steady-state conditions for reliable estimates. The metabolic steady state is assumed to be present when constant plasma cholesterol concentration, unchanging fecal excretion of steroids, and constant body weight all coexist during long periods of study. Except for chromatographic balance, all methods estimate the daily 'endogenous cholesterol turnover' which is the amount of daily synthesis and absorption; therefore, they can directly estimate the daily synthesis only on cholesterol-free diets. When the diet contains cholesterol, the values for synthesis can be obtained by simultaneous measurement of absorption by any one of the methods described on page 47.

Sterol Balance Methods

Cholesterol balance is perhaps the most important concept developed for reliable studies on different parameters of cholesterol metabolism in man. The credit for the development and establishment of cholesterol balance methods goes to *Ahrens, Grundy*, and their associates at the Rockefeller University [178, 296]. Although cumbersome and difficult, these methods are the gold standards against which other methods are validated.

The cholesterol balance methods are based on the assumption that losses of endogenous cholesterol and its metabolites occur predominantly in the feces; therefore, on a cholesterol-free diet the amounts of cholesterol and its metabolites lost in the feces represent the net synthesis of cholesterol in the body. It is perhaps worth noting that between 50 and 100 mg of cholesterol is lost daily from the skin surface [36, 333, 334], and about 50 mg of cholesterol per day is converted to steroid hormones [61], the catabolites of which are lost in the urine. However, these amounts remain more or less constant in most abnormalities of lipid transport. The excretory products of cholesterol in the feces can be estimated either by the use of isotopes or by the use of TLC and GLC. The details of the combined isotopic and chromatographic methods for estimation of dietary cholesterol, fecal neutral, and acidic steroids are given on page 125–132. Only the theoretical basis underlying these methods will be given in this section.

Isotopic Balance Method

The isotopic balance method was introduced by *Hellman et al.* [199]. This method involves an i.v. injection of radioactive cholesterol to label plasma cholesterol, and then waiting for a few days until the SA of plasma cholesterol comes to an equilibrium with the SA of biliary cholesterol and biliary acids. However, estimates of fecal steroids are more reliable if one waits 4–6 weeks for complete equilibration among various miscible pools before beginning the studies.

It was assumed by *Hellmann et al.* [199] that after a few days of equilibration, SA of plasma cholesterol equals the SA of biliary cholesterol and biliary bile acids. Although the SA values of plasma and biliary cholesterol are indeed similar, the SA of biliary bile acids remain somewhat greater than the SA of biliary or plasma cholesterol. This is due to the fact that the newly formed bile acids recirculate many times before being finally lost in the feces, whereas about half of the biliary cholesterol entering the duodenum is lost in a single transit during enterohepatic circulation.

Since it is the biliary and not the fecal cholesterol which has SA identical to that of plasma cholesterol, and since it relates to the time the cholesterol is first secreted into the bile, it is necessary to determine the exact (transit) time it takes for the biliary cholesterol to appear in the feces. The transit time is best determined by markers such as carmine red. After administration of about 300 mg of carmine red in a capsule, the time taken for the bulk of the dye to appear in the feces is the transit time. The SA of fecal cholesterol is then assumed to be equal to the SA of plasma cholesterol at a point in time earlier than the fecal collection with a lag equal to the transit time. The rate of decline in plasma cholesterol SA 5–6 weeks after the i.v. injection of radioactive cholesterol is so small that a few hours difference in the transit time makes little difference in the results. Therefore, investigators have generally assumed 36–48 h to be the transit time without actually determining it in all subjcts. However, the determination of the transit time is so simple that it is worth determining in every case.

Total fecal metabolites of endogenous cholesterol (mg/day)
= total fecal radioactivity (dpm/day) ÷ SA of plasma cholesterol (dpm/mg) at the time when these sterols were secreted into duodenum.

Such calculations are generally adequate for determining the total amounts of endogenous cholesterol (and its metabolites) which are lost in the feces per day. On a cholesterol-free diet, this will equal the amounts of cholesterol synthesized per day. Such calculations, however, do not give any idea as to how much endogenous cholesterol is lost as bile acids and how much as cholesterol. In order to determine the amounts of fecal bile acids and fecal neutral steroids, the fecal pools are extracted separately for neutral and acidic steroids, and calculations are made as follows:

Fecal neutral steroids of endogenous origin (mg/day)
= total radioactivity in neutral steroid fraction (dpm/day) ÷ SA of plasma cholesterol (dpm/mg) at 't' hours previously where 't' is transit time in hours.

These early calculations based on the assumptions of *Hellman et al.* [199], have since been refined and made more accurate by *Ahrens, Grundy*, and their associates at Rockefeller University as shown below.

In order to correct variations in fecal flow, the subjects are given chromic oxide daily in divided doses. Since it is neither degraded nor absorbed in the intestinal tract, its fecal recovery is used to correct variations in fecal flow. It was demonstrated that in most subjects given chromic oxide the fecal excretion begins to equal the daily intake at about 2 weeks after the start of its intake and remains so thereafter. Unfortunately, there are rare individuals (who are labeled non-ideal excretors) in whom this does not occur [105].

In addition to variations in fecal flow and the need for correcting it, *Grundy et al.* [179] after their extensive and meticulous investigations, came to the conclusion that a variable fraction of unabsorbed neutral sterols in the large gut is degraded by the intestinal bacteria to products no longer ex-tracted as neutral steroids. According to these authors, the fractions of unabsorbed cholesterol and dietary β-sitosterol degraded in the intestinal tract were identical. Furthermore, the degraded fraction remained more or less constant in a given individual, but it varied markedly from one subject to the next. They advised, therefore, that the amounts of fecal neutral steroids must be corrected for the losses due to degradation to obtain an accurate estimate of unabsorbed cholesterol. Since dietary β-sitosterol is not absorbed to any significant extent ($<5\%$), and since its degradation is identical to the degradation of unabsorbed cholesterol, *Grundy et al.* recommended that β-sitosterol should be used as a marker for evaluating cholesterol degradation in the intestinal tract [176, 179].

According to the methods outlined by *Grundy et al.* [179], the estimation of dietary β-sitosterol requires chromatographic techniques which are not ordinarily available in most laboratories. The percent degradation of dietary β-sitosterol can also be determined by giving a known amount of radioactive β-sitosterol orally (e.g. 5 μCi of ^{3}H-β-sitosterol if endogenous cholesterol is labeled with ^{14}C, or 2 μCi of ^{14}C-β-sitosterol if endogenous cholesterol is labeled with ^{3}H), and then calculating the fecal recovery in the next 8 days.

Thus, the current equation is:

Fecal neutral streoids of endogenous origin (mg/day)
= total radioactivity in the neutral steroid fraction (dpm/day)
$\div$ SA of plasma cholesterol (dpm/mg) at 't' hours previously
$\times$ correction for variation in fecal flow, and
$\times$ correction for degradation.

Studies conducted in our laboratory as well as other laboratories indicated that in patients receiving solid food diets (as against liquid formula diets consumed by patients studied by *Ahrens, Grundy*, and their associates), there is little if any degradation of unabsorbed neutral steroids [110, 237, 247, 248].

The corresponding equation for determination of fecal bile acids is:

Fecal bile acids (mg/day) = total radioactivity in acidic steroid fraction (dpm/mg)
$\div$ SA of plasma cholesterol 'U' hours previously
$\times$ correction for variation in fecal flow,

where 'U' hours refer to the time when plasma cholesterol had the SA equal to the SA of fecal bile acids, which may be taken as 56 h (see below).

As indicated earlier, the SA of biliary or fecal bile acids is generally greater than the corresponding SA of biliary or fecal cholesterol. Therefore, going back to the 36–48 h (usually assumed transit time) will not be adequate. *Grundy and Ahrens* [176] suggested that one should go back to 72–144 h. Studies done in our laboratories indicated that the SA of fecal bile acids was the same as the SA of plasma cholesterol, on average, 56 h before the mid-point in collection of 3-day fecal pools [247, 248].

On cholesterol-free diets, all fecal neutral and acidic steroids are derived from cholesterol synthesized in the body. Therefore, on cholesterol-free diets:

Cholesterol synthesis (mg/day) = fecal neutral steroids (mg/day) + fecal acidic steroids (mg/day); all corrected for variations in fecal flow and possible degradation of neutral steroids in the large gut.

When the diet contains cholesterol, the fecal neutral and acidic steroids are derived not only from the synthesized cholesterol, but also from the absorbed dietary cholesterol. Thus, the sum of fecal neutral and acidic steroids derived from endogenous cholesterol reflect the total turnover of cholesterol which equals the amounts synthesized and the amount of dietary cholesterol absorbed per day.

The cholesterol synthesis can be calculated if the amount of dietary cholesterol absorbed per day is known (for details of calculation of cholesterol absorption refer to p. 48, method 2).

Dietary cholesterol absorbed (mg/day) = cholesterol intake (mg/day) – unabsorbed dietary cholesterol (mg/day).
Unabsorbed dietary cholesterol (mg/day) = fecal total neutral steroids (mg/day) – fecal endogenous neutral steroids (mg/day).

Fecal total neutral steroids (mg/day) = total radioactivity in neutral steroids fraction (corrected for fecal flow variation and neutral steroid losses) (dpm/day) $\div$ SA of *fecal cholesterol* (dpm/mg).

The isotopic balance method has been validated and is in use in several laboratories.

Chromatographic Balance Method

In 1965, *Ahrens* and his associates developed chemical methods for the quantitative analysis of fecal neutral and acid steroids [178, 296]. This method involves the use of TLC and GLC; therefore, it is known as the chromatographic balance method. This method provides a quantitative and qualitative pattern of various conversion products of cholesterol, plant sterols and acidic steroids, and it can be used when the use of radioisotopes is contraindicated.

The chromatographic methods are particularly useful for estimating the intake and the fecal recovery of dietary β-sitosterol which are necessary for calculating degradation of neutral steroids in the intestinal tract.

One of the major advantages of a chromatographic balance method is the greater accuracy of estimating fecal bile acids.

The chromatographic method, however, is much more laborious and time-consuming than the isotope balance method. However, it was a major step forward in the studies on cholesterol balance in man.

On a cholesterol-containing diet, the fecal neutral steroids measured by chromatographic methods include cholesterol of endogenous origin as well as unabsorbed dietary cholesterol. Under these conditions, synthesis of cholesterol is calculated as follows:

Cholesterol synthesis (mg/day) = total fecal steroids (neutral and acidic) (mg/day) – cholesterol intake (mg/day).

Combined Isotopic and Chromatographic Balance Methods

When both isotopic and chromatographic balance methods are available, a simultaneous estimate of daily dietary cholesterol absorption can be obtained (for details, see p. 47, method 1). By the use of this method, the daily synthesis as well as turnover of cholesterol can be estimated [175].

Daily cholesterol turnover (mg/day) = fecal neutral steroids of endogenous origin (isotopic) (mg/day) + fecal acidic steroids (chromatographic) (mg/day).

This estimate of cholesterol turnover is better than that obtained by the use of isotopic methods alone since excretion of acidic steroids is determined with greater accuracy than by isotopic methods.

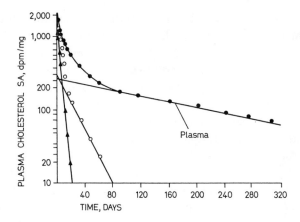

Fig. 8. Analysis of the decay of SA of plasma cholesterol (closed circles) based on the three-pool model. The terminal exponential portion of plasma cholesterol SA is extrapolated back to time 0. The difference between the observed SA values and the extrapolated line is represented by the open circles. Once again the terminal exponential portion of the slope of open circles is extrapolated back to time 0 and the difference between the slope of the open circles and the second extrapolated line is represented by the solid triangles.

Daily cholesterol synthesis (mg/day) = daily cholesterol turnover (mg/day) – daily absorption of exogenous cholesterol (mg/day).

The details for the isolation, purification, and quatitative of fecal steroids are given on pages 125–132.

Kinetic Analysis of Plasma Cholesterol SA-Time Curves

The body pools and turnover of (exchangeable) cholesterol in man can also be evaluated by techniques which are much simpler than the balance methods. They involve a single intravenous injection of labeled cholesterol and the determination of SA of plasma cholesterol at intervals for many months. The plasma cholesterol SA is plotted semilogarithmically (fig. 8), and the decay curves are analyzed mathematically. Two different approaches have been taken for their analysis: (1) compartmental analysis, assuming that the rate of disappearance of the tracer can be rationalized by one-, two-, or three-pool models, and (2) the input, output analysis which does not require curve fitting or the assumption of pools.

These approaches depend on two basic assumptions. (1) That the size of the total exchangeable pool of cholesterol does not change, and (2) that the entry of new unlabeled cholesterol (synthesized and dietary absorbed) into body pools remains constant during the long period of study. An increase in the size of body pools or a decrease in the rate of synthesis will cause the slope of decay of SA of plasma cholesterol to decrease, or if either factor (pool size or synthesis) changes in the other direction the decay of SA will be accelerated. In general, the use of SA time curves for collecting cholesterol turnover requires less effort than does the sterol balance methods. However, it takes many months to obtain accurate results; it may require as long as a year. On a cholesterol-containing diet, the synthesis of cholesterol cannot be calculated without knowledge of the dietary cholesterol and its percent absorption (p. 47). These methods give the rate constants for the removal of cholesterol from and the exchange of cholesterol between the pools, as well as the sizes of pools. However, it should be possible to assess the effects of pharmacological, physiological, and dietary manipulations on the sizes of rapidly exchangeable and (also possibly of) the slowly exchangeable pools.

Compartmental Analysis
One-Pool Model
This method was proposed by *Chobanian et al.* [85]. The assumption on which their calculations were based has since been found to be invalid. Comparison of this method with the sterol balance method has shown that the turnover values obtained on the basis of a one-pool model were on an average 65% higher [176]. This method now is of historic interest only.

Two-Pool Model
The theoretical basis and mathematical equations underlying this type of compartmental analysis were first proposed by *Tait et al.* [469] and *Gurpide et al.* [182, 183] for the study of steroid hormones. *Goodman and Noble* [166] applied these principles for the study of cholesterol metabolism. Originally, *Goodman and Noble* [166] used this method to calculate the turnover of cholesterol rate constants and the size of rapidly exchangeable pools. However, making certain assumptions, *Nestel et al.* [328] used the method to determine the lower and upper limits of the slowly exchangeable pools. *Grundy and Ahrens* [176] and subsequently *Sodhi and Kudchodkar* [431] compared this method with the sterol balance method and found that values obtained for cholesterol turnover were on an average 15% higher by this method as compared to the sterol balance method. Subsequent work in many other laboratories supported the above findings. *Wilson* [500] validated the method in baboons by comparing it with the results obtained by the isotopic

steady-state balance method, and also by actual determination of the mass of exchangeable cholesterol in various tissues. He showed that the total exchangeable cholesterol determined by the carcass analysis agreed closely with the total of the two exchangeable pools estimated from analysis of the decay curve. *Wilson*'s work showed that non-exchangeable cholesterol was not limited to the central nervous system as was previously believed [82, 85]. He found that to a varying degree tissues such as bone, skin, and muscle contain cholesterol which is essentially non-exchangeable. The readily exchangeable pool accounted for most of the cholesterol present in plasma, RBC, liver, small intestines, lung, spleen, kidney, and pancreas. By the same definition, a considerable fraction of cholesterol in other organs also belonged to the readily exchangeable pool, although the bulk of the slowly exchangeable pool was present in the same tissues, e. g. muscle, skin, bone, and adipose tissue. *Wilson*'s work showed that most tissues contain cholesterol belonging to both 'readily' as well as the 'slowly' exchangeable pools. It is worth bearing in mind that the definition of the pools is based on the rates of equilibration of the SA between plasma and tissues, and anatomical or physiological counterparts to these concepts do not exist. The function of these assumed models is only to facilitate the mathematical interpretation of the data, and possibly to compare these data obtained in different groups or under different experimental conditions.

Three-Pool Model (fig. 8, 9)

In 1970, *Samuel and Perl* [392] reported that in some patients (studied for a very long period) the linear portion of the decay curve deviates from monoexponential behavior after approximately 20–25 weeks. There was a flattening of the slope of the decay curve at that time. The same was seen by *Goodman et al.* [167], and they agreed that such data conformed to and can be satisfactorily resolved by a three-pool model.

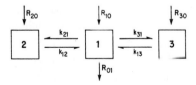

Fig. 9. Three-pool model of cholesterol turnover. The input and output is assumed to occur only from pool 1.

The appearance of the third exponential is explained by the existence of a poorly exchanging pool of significant size with very slow turnover. In a comparative study, it was found by *Goodman et al.* [167] that the three-pool model provided a significantly better description of the turnover curve than did the two-pool model. The values for cholesterol turnover obtained by the three-pool model were 8–9% lower than those obtained by the two-pool model, and they were closer to the values obtained by sterol balance techniques. The values obtained for rapidly exchangeable pools by both methods are similar. But, those obtained for the total exchangeable body of cholesterol by the two-pool method were significantly lower and unreliable. For a more accurate determination of cholesterol turnover and pool sizes, the isotope kinetic study should be carried out for at least 45 weeks, and the decay curve should be resolved into a three-pool model. As a result, the three-pool model will be discussed in detail.

As pointed out earlier, the pools have no physiological meaning and are merely mathematical constructs. In a three-pool model, it is assumed that the various tissue pools of exchangeable body cholesterol fall into three groups in terms of rates at which their SA equilibrates with that of plasma cholesterol. Pool 1 consists of cholesterol in fairly rapid equilibrium with plasma cholesterol. Pool 2 consists of cholesterol which equilibrates at an intermediate rate with plasma cholesterol, and pool 3 comprises that cholesterol which equilibrates with plasma cholesterol at a very slow rate. As discussed above, *Wilson* has shown that every tissue in the body may have cholesterol which may fall into more than one or two pools.

Such an analysis involves the labeling of plasma cholesterol by a single i.v. injection of a known amount of radioactive cholesterol. This can be achieved by anyone of the methods described on page 39. Fasting blood samples are obtained at 1, 2, 3, 5, and 7 days, then at weekly intervals for a period of at least 40–52 weeks. It is essential to measure the injected radioactivity precisely, and to obtain at least one blood sample during the first 3 days.

Plasma is separated from the blood and the SA of plasma cholesterol is determined. Time versus SA is then plotted on a semilogarithmic graph paper and curve fitting is done. Curve fitting can be done visually and the data can be analyzed manually. Similarly, both can be done better and more easily by the use of digital computers. Visual fitting of the exponential curve is subject to errors and bias of the investigator. The third exponential is obtained by extrapolation of the final linear portion to zero time. To obtain the second exponential, the difference between the experimental values and the values obtained after extrapolation of the terminal linear portion of the curve to zero time is replotted. On doing so, a new, second curve is generated. Extrapolation of the terminal linear portion of this second curve to zero time gives the second exponential. The first exponential is obtained exactly as described above, except that the plot is obtained using values of the second, newly generated curve (fig. 8).

The proposed three-pool model for cholesterol turnover is shown in figure 9 [167]. The method is based on the mathematical equations presented by *Skinner et al.* [422] which were adapted by *Goodman et al.* [167] for the calculation of cholesterol turnover. For this model, the equation of SA of pool 1 (a_1) is:

$$\frac{da_1}{dt} = k_{11}a_1 + \frac{M_2}{M_1}k_{12}a_2 + \frac{M_3}{M_1}k_{13}a_3$$

or

$$a_1 = A_1 e^{-a_1 t} + A_2 e^{-a_2 t} + A_3 e^{-a_3 t},$$

where k_{11} is the rate constant for the total rate of removal of cholesterol from pool 1, k_{12}, and k_{13} are the rate constants for the transfer of cholesterol from pools 2 and 3, respectively, into pool 1. M_1, M_2, and M_3 are the sizes (in grams) of pools 1, 2, and 3. A_1, A_2, and A_3 are the Y intercept values of the three exponentials of the SA-time curve. a_1, a_2, and a_3 are the rate constants of the three exponentials that describe the exponential curve. The values of these constants are determined from the half-lives of the three exponentials, since:

$$a = Ln2/t\frac{1}{2} = 0.0693/t\frac{1}{2}.$$

In the proposed model, movement of cholesterol out of the body (R_{o1}), i.e. catabolism and excretion, is assumed to occur only by way of the tissue pools which comprise the rapidly exchanging pool 1. This assumption permits the interpretation that the production rate (PR) in pool 1 is equivalent to the total body turnover rate. Evidence in support of this interpretation has been reported by a number of workers [176, 500]. The turnover rate calculated by this method on a cholesterol-free diet is equivalent to the cholesterol synthesis. If the diet contains appreciable amounts of cholesterol, then the turnover rate (PR) comprises both the newly biosynthesized cholesterol as well as the absorbed cholesterol. PR is described by general equations.

$$PR = \frac{R^*}{\int_0^\infty \sum_{i=1}^{nc} A_i e^{-a_i t} dt} = \frac{R^*}{\sum_{i=1}^{nc} \frac{A_i}{a_i}},$$

where R^* is the amount of radioactivity injected. The values for the rate constants for transfer between pools and the size of rapidly exchangeable pools can be calculated as follows:

$$M_1 = \frac{R^*}{A_1 + A_2 + A_3},$$

where M_1 = size (grams of rapidly exchangeable pool).

The rate constants are denoted by k, k_{11}, k_{22}, k_{33} = rate constants (day^{-1}) for the total rate of removal of cholesterol from pool 1, pool 2, and pool 3, respectively. k_{12} = Rate of transfer (day^1) of cholesterol from pool 2 to pool 1, and k_{13} = the rate of transfer (day^1) of cholesterol from pool 3 to pool 1 assuming that there is no direct excretion of cholesterol from pool 2 and pool 3:
then

$k_{12} = k_{22} \quad k_{13} = k_{33}$
$d_1 = k_{22} + k_{33} = a_2 + a_3 + (a_1{-}a_2)(A_2M_1) + (a_1{-}a_3)(A_3M_1)$
$d_2 = k_{22}k_{33} = (a_2{-}a_1)(a_2{-}a_3)A_2M_1{-}a_2^2 + d_1a_2$
$d_3 = k_{11} = a_1 + a_2 + a_3{-}d_1$
$d_4 = k_{13}k_{31} + k_{12}k_{21} = d_2 + d_3d_1{-}a_1a_2{-}a_2a_3{-}a_3a_1$
$d_5 = k_{13}k_{22}k_{31} + k_{12}k_{33}k_{21} = {-}a_1a_2a_3 + d_3d_2,$

then

$k_{11} = d_3$
$k_{12} = k_{22} = (-d_1 + \sqrt{d_1^2{-}4d_2})/2$
$k_{13} = k_{33} = (-d_1 - \sqrt{d_1^2{-}4d_2})/2$
$k_{21} = (d_5{-}d_4k_{22})/[(k_{33}{-}k_{22})k_{22}]$
$k_{31} = (d_4 k_{33}{-}d_5)/[(k_{33}{-}k_{22})k_{33}].$

k_{21} and k_{31} represent rate constants for the transfer of cholesterol from pool 1 to pool 2 and from pool 1 to 3, respectively.

Precise values for the two slowly exchangeable pools M_2 and M_3 cannot be obtained. However, upper and lower limiting values for M_2 (size of grams of pool 2) and M_3 (size in grams of pool 3) can be calculated making certain assumptions about the relative extent of synthesis of cholesterol in the tissues which comprise 1, 2, and 3; i.e. about the relative values of R_{10} (synthesis of cholesterol in pool g/day), R_{20} (synthesis of cholesterol in pool 2 g/day) and R_{30} (synthesis of cholesterol in pool 3 g/day).

Thus, the lower limiting value of M_2 is obtained when R_{20} = O. Lower limiting values for M_2

$= (R_{20} + M_1k_{21})/k_{22}$
$= M_1k_{21}/k_{22}$ when R_{20} = 0.

The upper limitating value for M_2 is obtained when R_{20} is at its maximal value. Since $R_{10} + R_{20} + R_{30} = PR$ and since PR represents the sum of endogenously synthesized cholesterol and dietary absorbed cholesterol, the maximal value for R_{20} can be estimated as PR – amount of dietary cholesterol absorbed. This is based on the assumption that all the newly absorbed cholesterol enters pool 1. Thus, the upper limiting for value $M_2 = (X + M_1k_{21})/k_{22}$, where $X = PR$ – amounts of dietary cholesterol absorbed.

Similarly, lower limiting value for M_3

$$= (R_{30} + M_1k_{31})/k_{33}$$
$$= M_1k_{31}/k_{33} \text{ when } R_{30} = 0,$$

and the upper limiting value for M_3

$$= (X + M_1k_{31})/k_{33}.$$

The minimal value for the total body exchangeable cholesterol (M) is obtained when $PR = R_{10}$ (R_{20} and R_{30} both equal zero).

$M = (M_1 + M_2\min + M_3\min)$. The maximal value for M is represented by $M = (M_1 + M_2\min + M_3\max)$ where the largest of the three compartments (pool 3) is at its upper limiting value. Rapidly exchangeable pool (M_1) can be subdivided into Mp and Mt. Mp = Amount of cholesterol (grams) only in plasma = plasma volume × concentration of cholesterol in plasma (mg/ml). Mt = Amount of cholesterol (grams) contained in other tissues comprising the rapidly exchangeable pool = M_1–Mp. Plasma volume is calculated assuming 4.5% of the body weight [125].

MCR, the metabolic clearance rate of cholesterol from pool 1 can be calculated as:

$$MCR = \frac{PR}{M_p}$$

However, valid the three -pool model may be as an overall approximation of the complex and dynamic state in the living animal, it should be emphasized that the body is actually comprised of a large number of individual compartments, each with its own turnover and exchange rates and sources of cholesterol. The overall model has meaning only because the major components of pools 1, 2, and 3 constitute a large fraction of the overall tissue cholesterol. Consequently, certain reservations must be kept in mind that changes in individual tissues may not necessarily be reflected in gross shifts in the sizes of exchangeable pools, just as alterations in serum concentration do not necessarily reflect changes in overall cholesterol balance [500].

Input-Output Analysis

Another approach for the analysis of the decay curves of plasma cholesterol SA was suggested by *Perl and Samuel* [355] in 1969. This mathematical approach is called the 'input-output' analysis, and is based on the theorems of *Stewart* [450] and *Hamilton et al.* [190]. This approach is made possible by the experimental findings that over most of the decay curves the SA of plasma cholesterol approximates the SA of cholesterol in the feces; the major route for cholesterol excretion. The decay curve then approximates a first passage indicator-dilution curve for which the 'input-output' method of analysis was designed. The application of 'input-output' analysis to the decay curve yields the following parameters: (1) Input rates (I^T) = sum of absorbed dietary and biosynthesized cholesterol (cholesterol turnover g/day) on a cholesterol-free diet. I_T = cholesterol synthesis (g/day). (2) Rapidly exchangeable mass (grams) of cholesterol (Ma). (3) Minimum value for the total exchangeable body mass (grams) of cholesterol, M). In calculating this minimum value for M it is assumed that cholesterol input occurs only into the rapidly exchangeable mass (Ma). (4) The remaining exchangeable mass (grams) of cholesterol (M-Ma), a minimum value for the slowly turning over exchangeable masses of cholesterol in the body.

Contrary to the compartmental analysis in which the number of pools should correspond to the number of exponentials revealed, input-output analysis is independent of the number of exponentials. Thus, the main difference between compartmental and input-output analysis is that the latter does not require the interpretations of a multiexponential curve in terms of discrete body pools of cholesterol. Input-output analysis utilizes only the area and the first time moment (mean transient time of tracer cholesterol or the 'center of gravity' of the area under the curve) of the plasma decay curves. It does not yield the intercompartmental exchange rates. It is applicable to the decay curves of a more general shape than those that can be fitted by a small number of exponentials; e.g. if more than three exponentials are observed, compartmental analysis cannot be used without involving the concept of additional discrete pools, whereas input-output analysis can be used without making any changes in assumptions [393].

It was found by *Samuel and Lieberman* [393] that the most accurate analysis of I^T (cholesterol turnover) is obtained if the studies are carried out for at least 45–50 weeks. To reduce the inconvenience and labor involved in such a long study, the authors have put forward a simplified method in which the plasma cholesterol SA is measured as infrequently as once a month. In short, this method involves the labeling of plasma cholesterol by a single i.v. injection of radioactive cholesterol and thereafter, frequent (4–6 moret blood samples are obtained during the first 2 weeks (the first datum poin) should be taken no later than 72 h after the tracer injection). For the following 40 weeks, blood is taken only once a month, and for the last 4 weeks of the experiment samples are obtained weekly or twice weekly. Plasma cholesterol SA is determined (p. 42) and the results expressed as percent dose of radioactivity given per gram of total plasma cholesterol by the calculation: $100 \times SA$ (dpm/g total plasma cholesterol) divided by the injected dose (dpm) of radioactive cholesterol. Computation of the various parameters can be done manually or more easily using a computer.

Computation of parameters is done as follows:

$$I_t = 100 / \int_o^\infty w(t)\, dt,$$

where (w) denotes SA as percent of injected dose per gram cholesterol at times (t) days. The value of I_T is equivalent to the reciprocal area under the decay curves from time 0 to infinity. To calculate this, the decay curve is extrapolated back to time zero and forward to infinity.

The mean transit time, $\overline{tp}$ (days), of tracer cholesterol represents the first time moment of the decay curves, or the 'center of gravity' of the area under the curves (the point at which the area could be balanced).

$$tp = \int_o^\infty tw(t)\, dt / \int_o^\infty w(t)\, dt.$$

The minimum value for total exchangeable body mass of cholesterol (M) (grams):

$$M = I_T \overline{tp}.$$

The rapidly exchangeable mass of body cholesterol (Ma) (grams):

$$Ma = 100 / w(o).$$

This value is determined from the extrapolation of the decay curve (data points of the initial 2 weeks) back to time zero. The remaining exchangeable mass of body of cholesterol is obtained as the difference: M-Ma (grams). Input-output analysis can be used with any curve shape or duration of experiments and is simpler in concept than compartmental analysis.

Isotopic Steady-State Method

The concept of isotopic steady state was introduced in 1957 by *Morris et al.* [307]. Using this technique, these workers were able to calculate only the relative contributions of dietary and newly synthesized cholesterol to the plasma cholesterol. The method involves feeding radioactive cholesterol in constant amounts; isotopic steady state was presumed to be reached after some weeks when the SA of plasma cholesterol reaches a plateau despite continued feeding of radioactive cholesterol. At this time, all readily miscible pools of cholesterol are assumed to be in equilibrium with the plasma pool. Thus:

Cholesterol in plasma derived from absorbed cholesterol (%) =
plasma cholesterol SA (dpm/mg) × 100 ÷ dietary cholesterol SA (dpm/mg).

Using this isotopic steady-state method, *Grundy and Ahrens* [176] were able to calculate absolute amounts of absorbed dietary cholesterol which *Morris et al.* [307] had not done. The equations for the calculation of exogenous cholesterol absorption are given on page 51 (method 3). Since the absolute amounts of absorbed cholesterol and the proportion of the plasma cholesterol derived from absorbed cholesterol are known, the cholesterol turnover and cholesterol synthesis can be calculated as follows:

Cholesterol turnover (mg/day) = daily absorption of dietary cholesterol (mg/day) ÷ fraction of plasma colesterol derived from absorbed cholesterol.
Cholesterol synthesis (mg/day) = cholesterol turnover (mg/day) – daily absorption of dietary cholesterol (mg/day).

Quantitative estimation of absorbed cholesterol and cholesterol synthesis can also be made in isotopic steady-state methods in combination with an isotopic sterol balance or isotopic kinetics of plasma cholesterol SA analysis method. These approaches have been used by *Wilson and Lindsey* [501] and by *Wilson* [500] to study cholesterol metabolism in man and animals. The percentage of circulating cholesterol derived from dietary and from endogenous sources are estimated by an isotopic steady-state method. Cholesterol turnover is estimated either by use of an isotopic sterol balance method or by the analysis of plasma cholesterol SA decay curve. The daily absorption of dietary cholesterol and the daily synthesis of cholesterol are determined as follows:

Daily dietary cholesterol absorption (mg/day) = daily cholesterol turnover (mg/day) × fraction of plasma cholesterol derived from absorbed dietary cholesterol.
Daily cholesterol synthesis (mg/day) = daily cholesterol turnover (mg/day) – daily cholesterol absorbed (mg/day).

It may take a long time, possibly months, to obtain these results since they are valid only if the data are collected after an isotopic steady state has been obtained [361, 262].

Measurement of Cholesterol Synthesis in a Nonsteady State

The quantitative methods described above can be used for the measurement of cholesterol synthesis only under metabolic steady-state conditions. Absolute values for synthesis of cholesterol cannot be obtained in a metabolic nonsteady state, e.g. after treatment with hypolipidemic drugs. To overcome this problem, two new and simple methods have been proposed. Both methods are in early stages of evaluation, and if validated under different experimental conditions, they would be extremely useful in the study of cholesterol metabolism.

Measurement of Influx Rate of Newly Synthesized Cholesterol into Plasma

This method, developed by *Nestel and Kuchodkar* [326] measures the influx of newly synthesized cholesterol into plasma. It is based on the precursor product kinetics of plasma squalene and newly synthesized cholesterol during a 6- to 8-hour i.v. infusion of radioactive mevalonic acid. The method takes advantage of the fact that squalene, a precursor of cholesterol, is present in plasma in amounts that are readily measurable. During an infusion of radioactive mevalonate, the SA of plasma squalene reaches a plateau in about a couple of hours, and thus the rate at which newly formed labeled cholesterol is derived from squalene can be calculated as follows:

Newly synthesized cholesterol influx in plasma (mg/24 h) = rate of increase of FC radioactivity/h × 24 × plasma volume divided by the SA of squalene.

Several assumptions are made in this estimation: (1) squalene is an obligatory precursor of cholesterol; (2) the plasma squalene is in equilibrium with that pool of tissue squalene, especially in the liver, from which cholesterol is being synthesized, and (3) the efflux of rate of newly synthesized FC is substantially slower than the influx so that minimal radioactivity is lost from plasma during the period of study. This seems probable since the turnover of cholesterol (in the pool which includes plasma) has a half-time of 4–5 days.

In short, the method involves an i.v. infusion of radiomevalonate: One fifth of the solution is infused rapidly over 10 min and the remainder by constant i.v. infusion over 6–8 h. It was found that plasma squalene radioactivity became constant by 2 h, and that the rate of increase in plasma FC radioactivity was linear after the second hour up to the eighth hour. Blood samples are collected (15–20 ml) anytime between the second and eighth hours, and the concentration of and the radioactivity in squalene and FC are determined.

This method has not been compared with other established techniques using the same subjects. However, it was found that the influx rates of newly formed plasma FC in subjects eating normal amounts of cholesterol were comparable with those reported for the total body sterol synthesis obtained by sterol balance techniques [unpublished observations]. The influx rate was almost trebled with colestipol treatment and was reduced substantially on a high cholesterol diet and by clofibrate treatment as expected.

The method does not distinguish between the secretion of newly synthesized cholesterol into plasma, in lipoproteins, from that appearing in plasma due merely to isotopic exchange. The method, however, is useful in comparing conditions where rates of exchange are assumed to remain the same.

The method is simple and the results can be obtained within a day or two. A constant infusion of radioactive mevalonate and only 2–3 blood samples are needed. The test can be repeated frequently to study the effect of different regimens.

Measurement of Cholesterol Synthesis by Isotope Kinetics of Squalene

Another method recently proposed by *Liu et al.* [269] is also based on the isotope kinetics of plasma squalene. This procedure is simple, can be carried out in an outpatient clinic, and does not require a metabolic steady state. A single dose of each of ^{14}C-mevalonic acid and ^{3}H-cholesterol is given i.v., and SA of plasma squalene (^{14}C) and of plasma cholesterol (^{14}C and ^{3}H) are then determined. From the SA curves of the ^{14}C- and ^{3}H-cholesterol (expressed as percent dose per gram cholesterol), the percent conversion of ^{14}C-mevalonic acid to ^{14}C-cholesterol is determined, and from this the dose of ^{14}C-squalene entering cholesterol is estimated. The reciprocal of the area under the SA slope of ^{14}C-squalene when multiplied by the dose of ^{14}C-squalene, gives the rate of cholesterol synthesis if the following assumptions are made: (1) squalene is an obligatory precursor for cholesterol; (2) input of biosynthesized squalene equals cholesterol synthesis, and (3) the equilibrium between plasma squalene and metabolically active squalene in tissues is rapid.

In four studies carried out by the authors [269], the rates of cholesterol synthesis determined by this technique compared favorably with the results obtained by the balance methods conducted simultaneously. This method, although rapid compared to other established methods, requires at least 5–6 weeks to obtain reliable results. However, the method, if validated, will be very useful for studies on cholesterol metabolism in man. Recently, these

workers [288] have shown that percent conversion of mevalonate to cholesterol is directly related to the synthesis of cholesterol as measured by sterol
balance techniques in different metabolic conditions.

There are some theoretical questions which may have to be resolved.
It has generally been believed that most, if not all, of the mevalonate is
ultimately incorporated into cholesterol. Differences in the rates of cholesterol synthesis, according to the current ideas, may influence the time it take
for mevalonate to be converted to cholesterol, but not its proportion. However, this may or may not be true.

A second question relates to the differences in the metabolism of labeled
cholesterol made from the mevalonate and the labeled cholesterol injected
as a suspension. It has been shown that immediately after the i.v. injections
of radioactive mevalonate and radioactive cholesterol in alcoholic saline, the
losses from the body of cholesterol synthesized from mevalonate may be
somewhat greater than those for radioactive cholesterol injected as a suspension [439, 440]. However, the difference in the metabolism of the cholesterol derived from the two sources while biologically significant may be quite
unimportant quantitatively.

Qualitative Methods

The above methods can give absolute values of cholesterol turnover or
cholesterol synthesis. Other more simple methods are available to assess the
relative rates of cholesterol synthesis. These qualitative methods are useful
for comparing two experimental conditions in the same subject (e.g. effects
of drug therapy or various dietary manipulations) or possibly between different groups of subjects. The usefulness of these methods in comparing
two individuals is unsubstantiated.

Relative Rates of Acetate and Mevalonate Incorporation into Plasma FC

This method is based on rationale that only a very small fraction of the
acetate pool enters the pathway of cholesterol synthesis and that the site of
its control is between acetate and mevalonate. Once acetate is converted to
mevalonate, most of it must inevitably go into synthesis of cholesterol. The
rate of acetate conversion into mevalonate then in fact determines the rate of
cholesterol synthesis. The sizes of precursors pool of acetate and mevalonate
are so small and their turnover rates so rapid that they do not significantly
alter the proportion of administered radioactive acetate or mevalonate going

into cholesterol except by the ambient rates of conversion of acetate and mevalonate to cholesterol.

This method was developed independently by *Miettinen* [291] and *Sodhi et al.* [436]. It involves an i.v. injection of a mixture of acetate-1-^{14}C and mevalonate-2-^{3}H in a known proportion, and the determination of the ratio of the two isotopes in plasma FC between 3 and 4 h (at peak SA of FC) after the injection. The ratio estimated only in one sample or alternatively an average of the ratios in 2 or 3 samples (taken during this time) may be taken. In theory, these results should be influenced to greater or lesser degree by the sizes of precursor pools of acetate and mevalonate, and by the rates of hepatic synthesis of cholesterol. Despite the absence of definite information about sizes of precursor pools of acetate and mevalonate in different experimental conditions, the results obtained by this method are in accord with those obtained by the sterol balance methods, or by the analysis of decay curves of plasma cholesterol SA [433]. Results obtained by *Miettinen* [292] also indicate that the method provides a reasonable index for evaluating the status of cholesterol synthesis *invivo*. Most of the recently synthesized cholesterol in plasma 2–4 h after the injection of radioactive precursors comes from the liver and therefore these ratios reflect the activity of this organ and not of the entire body.

Serum Squalene and Methyl Sterols

It was proposed by *Miettinen* [291] that quantitation of serum squalene and unesterified methyl sterols may be used as indicators of cholesterol synthesis *in vivo*. It is assumed that during the synthesis of cholesterol in liver some precursors leak out of the liver into plasma. The concentrations of these precursors of cholesterol in plasma reflect the rates of their synthesis, and thus the synthesis of cholesterol in the liver. *Miettinen* [291, 292] was the first to use this method by estimating dihydrolanosterol, methosterols, mono-unsaturated dimethylsterols, diunsaturated dimethylsterols, and lanosterols.

The method involves extraction of approximately 10 ml of plasma by chloroform-methanol, separation of unesterified methyl sterols and squalene by TLC and their determination by GLC.

It was found by *Miettinen* [293] that the concentration of unesterified methyl sterols in serum did not correlate well with cholesterol synthesis as determined by the sterol balance technique. This might have been due to the disproportionate binding of these methyl sterols to different plasma lipoproteins. However, it was found that the expression of unesterified methyl sterol concentration in relation to the concentration of FC in plasma eliminated the effect of an altered lipoprotein level on unesterified methyl sterol concentration and gave a better measure of cholesterol production. Thus, it was found that the ratios of methyl sterols to FC were raised in conditions in which the cholesterol synthesis were increased and vice versa. Recently, a number of workers [250, 269, 326, 400] have shown that the concentration of plasma squalene accurately reflects the state of cholesterol synthesis. Thus, it has been shown that concentrations of plasma squalene rise significantly when cholesterol synthesis is stimulated by treatment with cholestyramine, colestipol, carbohydrate, etc., and fall in conditions which are known to inhibit cholesterol synthesis, i.e. high cholesterol diets, fasting, and nicotinic acid treatment.

Ahrens and his associates [269] have recently described a simple, accurate and reproducible method for the estimation of squalene in plasma and other tissues. In this method, a known amount of squalane (a recovery standard) is added to 4–5 ml plasma and it is saponified at 70 °C for 2 h after adding 10 ml of methanolic-KOH (final concentration of KOH 10% w/v). The non-saponifiable fraction is extracted with 20 ml of PE (BP 30–60 °C), and after its concentration is transferred to an 8 × 1 cm alumina column. Squalene and squalane are then eluted with 50 ml PE, concentrated and quantitated by GLC. GLC is carried out using a gas chromatograph equipped with hydrogen flame ionization detector; using a 6-feet column of 1% dexsil 300 on 100–200 mesh Supelcoport. Temperature of column, flash heater and detector are held at 235, 265, and 255 °C, respectively, and nitrogen is used as a carrier gas with an inlet pressure of 30 psi. Squalene in sample is calculated as follows:

$$\text{Squalene in sample } (\mu g) = \frac{\text{squalene area}}{\text{squalane area}} \times \mu g \text{ squalane added.}$$

Determination of Hepatic 3-Hydroxy-3-Methyl-Glutaryl-CoA Reductase (HMG-CoA Reductase Activity)

The rate-determining step in biosynthesis of cholesterol is the formation of mevalonic acid from 3-hydroxy-3-methyl glutaryl-CoA. This reaction is catalyzed by the microsomal enzyme 3-hydroxy-3-methyl glutaryl-CoA reductase (HMG-CoA reductase EC 1.1.134). It has been well established that the activity of this enzyme accurately reflects the state of cholesterol synthesis [22, 72, 375, 415].

The enzyme has been studied extensively in experimental animals. Its use in humans, however, is limited by the necessity of obtaining fresh liver biopsy specimens which may or may not always be possible.

Nicolau et al. [330] have recently described an assay for the determination of hepatic HMG-CoA reductase in man. The method described below for the assay of HMG-CoA reductase utilizes the techniques of *Mosbach, Shefer,* and their associates for the preparation of liver microsomes and their incubations [330, 331, 406] and that of *Goldfarb and Pitot* [160] and of *Ackerman et al.* [3] for the extraction and quantitation of mevalonate.

Preparation of Liver Microsomes. Hepatic tissue sample is obtained by percutaneous liver biopsy. Between 20 and 60 mg tissue is removed by Menghini's technique utilizing a 16-gauge Menghini needle. To eliminate the effect of possible diurnal variation in the activity, hepatic HMG-CoA reductase sampling is done at a fixed time during the 24-hour cycle. After removal, the tissue is immediately placed in an ice-cold solution (for homogenization) which is composed of sucrose (0.3 M), nicotinamide (0.075 M), EDTA (0.002 M), and mercaptoethanol (0.02 M). All further manipulations are done at 4 °C. The liver tissue is blotted dry on a sterile gauze and weighed. The tissue is then transferred into a 15-ml centrifuge tube and homogenized with a loose-fitting teflon pestle (radial clearance of 0.5 mm). The procedure is standardized by employing a motor driven pestle at 1,500 rpm and homogenizing for 10–15 sec with four up and down excursions of the pestle, taking care to avoid excessive cellular disruption. Homogenizing medium is then added to obtain a 5–10% homogenate (w/v).

The homogenate is then centrifuged at 11,000 g for 10 min to sediment nuclei, cell debris, and mitochondrial fractions. The supernatant solution is transferred into a 4-ml polycarbonate tube and centrifuged at 100,000 g for 60 min. The supernatant solution is decanted and the pellet containing microsomes is washed with 1 ml of homogenizing medium and centrifuged again (100,000 g for 60 min). The supernatant solution is decanted and the microsomal pellet is homogenized in the same centrifuge tube with a volume of homogenizing medium to give a solution of known concentration (to contain between 1 and 3 mg protein per 1 ml).

Incubation. Incubation of the microsomes is carried out in 15-ml culture tubes in air at 37 °C in a shaking water bath for 30 min. The assay system, in a total volume of 0.85 ml, contains phosphate buffer pH 7.2, 100 mM; MgCl$_2$, 3 mM; NADP, 3 mM; glucose-6-phosphate, 10 mM; glucose-6-phosphate dehydrogenase (EC 1.1.149), 3 enzyme units; mercaptoethanol 20 mM; R-S-[3-^{14}C]-HMG-CoA, 0,4 mM, and microsomal protein 0.1–0.4 mg.

Extractions and Quantitation of Mevalonate. A number of methods have been developed for the assay of this enzyme. Most assay methods involve the measurement of [14C]-mevalonate formed during incubation of [14C]-HMG-CoA with hepatic microsomes in the presence of NADPH or an NADPH-generating system. The product is extracted along with unreacted HMG-CoA and/or HMG and it is then subsequently purified by column [20, 122, 219], GLC [418] or TLC [160, 405]. *Goldfarb and Pitot's* [160] method circumvents the need for quantitative extraction of [14C]-mevalonate by using [3H]-mevalonate as an internal reference standard to determine the extraction efficiency. All these assay procedures, although reliable, accurate and sensitive, are time consuming. *Ackerman et al.* [3] have recently introduced a simple, rapid and accurate method for the extraction of mevalonate. The method is based on the fact that, in a slightly acidic (pH 6.7–6.9), saturated aqueous solution of an alkali metal salt, mevalonic acid is mainly present as mevalonolactone, whereas HMG is mainly present as the metal salt. The relative nonpolar mevalonolactone can be extracted into an organic phase, while the polar HMG salt and very polar HMG-CoA remain in the aqueous phase.

The Chloroform Extraction Assay. After the enzymatic reaction is stopped by addition of 1 ml of 2 N HCl, a known amount of [3H]-mevalonolactone is added to serve as an internal reference standard. The sample is allowed to stand for 30 min at room temperature to insure lactonization, and is then transferred to a counting vial with adequate rinses of buffer. Unlabeled mevalonolactone (10 mg) is added followed by the addition of 2.3 g of an equal molar mixture of solid K_2HPO4–KH_2PO4. Samples are then incubated with shaking (2 oscillations per sec) in a Dubnoff incubator at 37 °C for 37 min. 6 ml of chloroform is then added, followed by vigorous shaking of the mixture by hand for a few seconds. After releasing the pressure, the sample is shaken again and then filtered into a counting vial through a Whatman 1 PS phase separating filter paper which is first wetted with chloroform. The aqueous material from the filter paper is transferred back to the extraction vial and the chloroform extraction is repeated once again. To the combined chloroform filtrates, 1 ml of a saturated solution of equimolar K_2HPO4–KH_2PO4 is added and shaken vigorously. The contents are then filtered into a counting vial using a fresh 1 PS phase separating filter paaer made wet with chloroform. The chloroform filtrate is evaporated to dryness under a stream of nitrogen and the radioactivity is counted after adding water (0.5 ml) and 10 ml aquasol. A blank consisting of all assay material except the liver microsomes (or with boiled liver microsomes) is carried through a similar procedure. The [^{14}C]-radioactivity obtained in the blank sample is then subtracted from the [^{14}]C-radioactivity of the sample.

The chloroform sample extraction procedure recovers 50–60% of the mevalonate present in the incubation mixture. The [^{14}C]-radioactivity values of the sample therefore are corrected using the recovery of [^{3}H]-mevalonate added as the internal reference standard [160]. The activity of the enzyme is expressed as the moles of mevalonate formed/min/mg protein.

Turnover of Total Body and Plasma Cholesterol

It is worth noting that parameters of cholesterol metabolism determined by methods such as cholesterol balance and isotope kinetic analyses are absorption, synthesis and elimination of cholesterol from the system. As such they are directly relavent only to the turnover of total body (exchangeable) cholesterol (Figure 10a) and not to the turnover of plasma cholesterol (Figure 10b). The assumption is therefore made that changes in the total body cholesterol will "somehow" be reflected in the levels of plasma cholesterol. The validity of this critical assumption under all conditions has yet to be established.

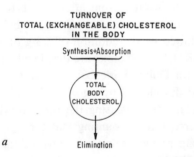

a

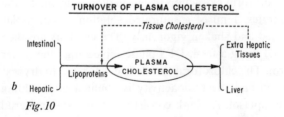

b

Fig. 10

Chapter VI. Esterification of Plasma Free Cholesterol

Of the total cholesterol in plasma, approximately $1/3$ is in the free form and the other $2/3$ are esterified [4, 64]. Under normal circumstances, the ratio of FC/esterified cholesterol in plasma remains remarkably constant [64]. The ratios can, however, be grossly distorted in liver disease or in genetic deficiency of enzyme which esterifies plasma FC [338, 413].

After a meal containing fats, cholesterol absorbed from intestinal lumen enters the circulation predominantly as CE. However, during postabsorptive or fasting state, most of the cholesterol entering the circulation comes from the liver, and it is believed to be predominantly in the free form [153, 154]. It was suggested by *Glomset* [154] that recently synthesized hepatic lipoproteins contain only the FC and CE in plasma are formed later while the lipoproteins are undergoing metabolic changes in the plasma compartment [154].

Sperry [442] was the first to observe that on incubating human plasma there was a progressive increase in plasma CE. In 1962, *Glomset* [152] presented evidence that the esterification of plasma FC is brought about by an enzyme in plasma which transfers the fatty acid at position 2 of lecithin to FC in the lipoproteins. The enzyme was named lecithin: cholesterol acyl transferase (LCAT).

The LCAT does not react equally with all plasma lipoproteins. Plasma HDL is the preferred substrate for its action [156]. In fact, the enzyme may be secreted by the liver along with HDL, and even in circulation it may exist as a HDL:enzyme complex. It is believed that the initial reaction of LCAT takes place on or within HDL molecules [154], thereby decreasing the content of FC in HDL. Other plasma lipoproteins are believed to transfer their FC to make up for the decline in the HDL FC. In this sense, the LCAT:HDL complex may be viewed as a single system which helps in the esterification of all plasma FC. Recent work of *David et al.* [104] suggests that VLDL may also act as a substrate for LCAT under certain *in vitro* conditions.

In addition to its enzymatic activity, LCAT is also believed to facilitate non-enzymatic transfers of lipids among lipoproteins. In exchange for CE from HDL, the plasma VLDL transfers triglycerides to HDL [329, 370].

Although these transfers have been demonstrated *in vitro*, their occurrence *in vivo* has yet to be established.

The physiological significance of esterification of plasma FC by LCAT is still unclear. Recently synthesized VLDL contain triglycerides in the core which is covered by a surface film made up of proteins, phospholipids, and FC [396, 522]. After they are secreted by the liver into plasma, there is a progressive loss of triglycerides from (the core of) VLDL leading to a progressive reduction in the size as well as in the surface area of the particles. This makes some of the surface film redundant, and the extra FC is converted to the CE presumably to increase the efficiency of transport in plasma [401]. According to this view, increase in the rate of metabolism of VLDL should be associated with increased activity of LCAT and, indeed, *Nestel et al.* [322, 325], as well as *Kudchodkar and Sodhi* [244], have shown that the rates of esterification of plasma FC are directly related to the turnover of both plasma VLDL and cholesterol. Similarly, *Rose and Juliano* [380] have shown that LCAT activity is increased during the absorptive phase, when plasma chylomicron concentration is high.

An earlier suggestion of *Glomset* [153, 154] that the function of LCAT was related to the transport of cholesterol from peripheral tissues to the liver has attracted considerable attention recently [297, 448], when it was suggested that HDL may transport tissue cholesterol into plasma for its transport to the liver for catabolism.

Methods to Study the Turnover of Plasma CE

The methods to study the turnover of plasma CE can be divided into three classes: (1) *in vivo*, (2) *in vitro*, and (3) *in vivo/in vitro* methods.

In vivo *Method*

After pulse labeling of FC in plasma, the SA of plasma CE begins to increase and it reaches a peak value in about 2–3 days, at which time the SA slope of CE is crossed by the declining SA of FC. Thereafter, the SA slopes of plasma FC and esterified cholesterol remain parallel: the SA of CE remaining slightly greater than that of FC, in accord with the precursor product relationship (fig. 11). *Nestel and Monger* [324] utilized these SA slopes of FC and CE to estimate the daily turnover of plasma CE. The model for determination was based on mathematical details outlined previously by *Zilversmit* [521].

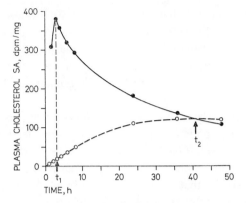

Fig. 11. The SA slopes of plasma FC (closed circles) and CE (open circles) after pulse labeling of plasma FC. The SA are plotted on a Cartesian graph paper to determine the fractional turnover rate of plasma CE. The difference between the SA values of CE at t_2 and t_1 is divided by the area enclosed between the two slopes from t_1 to t_2.

In this method, the plasma FC is labeled either by injecting radioactive precursors such as acetate or mevalonate, or by injecting radioactive cholesterol. i.v. Blood samples are withdrawn at frequent intervals, and the SA of plasma FC and esterified cholesterol is determined. The SA slopes of plasma FC and esterified choesterol are plotted on a Cartesian graph paper, and the fractional turnover rate (FTR) of CE is calculated as in the following equation (fig. 11):

$$FTR = \frac{SA\ (CE)\ t_2 - SA\ (CE)\ t_1}{Area\ enclosed\ by\ two\ slopes\ between\ t_1\ and\ t_2} \cdot$$

The t_1 and t_2 refer to the times chosen for the determination. *Nestel and Monger* [324] used the time of peak SA of FC and CE as t_1 and t_2. By determining the values of SA of plasma FC and esterified cholesterol at 1-hour intervals, *Barter* [24] showed that accurate results can be obtained anytime during the first 3–8 h after the i.v. injection of radioisotopes to label plasma cholesterol. Thus, it is not necessary to obtain blood samples for 3 days as was done by *Nestel and Monger* [324] and by us [244].

The following assumptions are made in this method: (1) FC in plasma or cholesterol pools in rapid equilibrium with plasma are the immediate precursors for plasma CE, and (2) the plasma CE constitute a single homogenous pool.

Nestel and Couzens [323] showed that for as long as 40 h after the mevalonic acid injection, the SA of liver CE was well below the SA of plasma CE, suggesting that hepatic CE were not major precursors of plasma esterified cholesterol. Furthermore, it has been demonstrated that in patients with familial deficiency of plasma LCAT the levels of plasma CE remain very low [338].

It has been shown that the turnover of CE in different classes of plasma lipoproteins is heterogenous. The FTR of CE within HDL is greater than that of CE in VLDL and LDL. *Nestel and Monger* [324] however, showed that the fractional turnover rates of whole plasma represent the average FTR of CE in different lipoproteins, and that the turnover rate in whole plasma equals the sum of separate turnover rates of CE in the different classes of plasma lipoproteins.

In vitro *Methods*

The best method for '*in vitro*' determination of plasma LCAT would be an immunochemical procedure which will determine the concentration of the enzyme in plasma. Such a method has recently been developed [486]. Its application for routine laboratory use, however, may be a few years away.

Several assay procedures and their modifications have been worked out to measure the LCAT activity *in vitro* [155, 284, 316, 351, 452, 489]. All these methods are based on the principle that LCAT which is present in plasma decreases the FC and at the same time increases the CE. Estimation of the changes in the concentration of FC and/or CE is therefore a measure of the LCAT activity. The changes in the concentration of plasma FC or CE are rather small, and are therefore difficult to measure accurately by conventional colorimetric methods. The changes (decrease in FC), however, can be measured accurately by GLC [47, 284] or by recently developed enzymatic methods [316, 351]. Alternatively, the formation of CE can be estimated by the use of plasma labeled with radioactive cholesterol [155, 452]. In this method, the FC of plasma is labeled with radioactive cholesterol taking care that the plasma CE are not labeled or labeled to a very small extent, any new formation of CE as a results of the action of the enzyme is readily detected by determining the increase in radioactivity occurring in the CE fraction. By increasing the SA of FC in the labeled plasma, the sensitivity of the method can be increased to such a level that even a few micrograms of high SA FC when converted to CE causes enough increase in the radioactivity of plasma CE to be measured accurately. The total amount of CE formed is calculated as follows: *μmole of CE formed/ml/h* = radioactivity in plasma CE (dpm/

ml) at the end of incubation – radioactivity in plasma CE (dpm/ml) at zero time $\div$ SA of FC (dpm/μmol) of the sample at zero time.

It should be noted that the precursor FC for the formation of CE may be on some special reactive sites on HDL although the experimental determination of SA are made on total FC present in plasma. It is therefore important to ensure that there is complete equilibration of SA of all FC in plasma lipoproteins.

The pros and cons of various methods of labeling plasma with radioactive cholesterol (p. 39) and the methods for the separation (p. 15) and quantitation (p. 24) of FC and CE have been given elsewhere in this book. Only points of relevance to the LCAT determination *in vitro* will be touched upon in this section.

In general, two types of assays are available for the measurement of LCAT activity: (1) the assays utilizing a heat-inactivated plasma as a common substrate source and a small amount of plasma ([0.1 to 0.5 ml] in which LCAT is to be measured) as an enzyme source [155], and (2) the assays in which autologous plasma serves as substrate as well as the source of enzyme [452].

The first method developed for the detection of LCAT activity was used by *Glomset and Wright* [155] to follow the activity of the enzyme during purification procedures. The method involved incubating a small volume of test plasma (enzyme source) for a few hours with an excess of heat-inactivated pooled plasma (common substrate) and an albumin stabilized emulsion of radioactive FC. The esterification of FC present in the mixture of substrate and test plasma was determined after isolating the sterols by TLC. If all FC in plasma is assumed to constitute a single pool of substrate, and if the substrate plasma is also assumed to be devoid of other activators and inhibitors of the reaction, then the activity of plasma LCAT determined in this system should be independent of the substrate source as long as the substrate was present in excess. However, when the same test plasma was used with different substrate plasmas, all of which were present in excess, the results differed markedly from one substrate to another [47]. Furthermore, when tested against another developed by *Stokke and Norum* [452] using autologous non-heated lipoproteins as substrates, results obtained by the two methods differed by as much as 100% [47].

The method used by *Stokke and Norum* [452] involves the stabilization of radioactive cholesterol in acetone in a solution of albumin, and complete evaporation of the acetone. The albumin stabilized radioactive cholesterol is then incubated with test plasma for 4 h to allow for equilibration of the radioactive FC with all the FC in plasma lipoproteins. To prevent esterification of radioactive FC during the period of equilibration, it is necessary to add inhibitors of the reaction to the preincubation mixture and a de-inhibitor is added just before the mixture is incubated to determine the activity of LCAT.

It was shown recently that the albumin used for stabilizing radioactive cholesterol may contain some LCAT activity which can be destroyed by heating the albumin solution at 60 °C for 30 min [489]. Furthermore, it has been demonstrated that for reproducible results complete evaporation of the acetone from the mixture containing albumin stabilized radioactive cholesterol is necessary.

It should be kept in mind that no *in vitro* method can mimic the conditions of rapidly turning over plasma lipoproteins *in vivo*. Constant supply of fresh substrate is nearly impossible to imitate *in vitro*. In early procedures to determine the LCAT activity, the plasma was generally incubated for many hours; the results of which obviously were influenced by availability of substrate in addition to the concentration of enzyme. Therefore, emphasis is now put on the initial rate of the reaction. Various studies have indicated that the initial rate of reaction is linear anywhere from 1 to 2 h and therefore the tendency has been to use periods of even less than 1 h. Such attempts are directed towards making the test more responsive to the enzyme concentrations than to the availability of substrate. However, the reaction occurs on plasma HDL, and it is conceivable that small amounts of HDL present in the test plasma may also participate in the initial reaction of LCAT (in the test plasma). Since the reaction is continued for at least up to a period of 40–60 min, the contributions of HDL in test plasma will be quantitatively insignificant.

Since the continued reaction of plasma LCAT is to a degree dependent on the transfers of lipids between different lipoproteins present in the mixture, it is desirable to use a method which does not denature any of the lipoproteins present in the substrate plasma. Furthermore, since the concentrations of lipids or lipoproteins in the reaction mixture may influence the LCAT reaction it is desirable to reproduce the *in vivo* conditions of the subject as closely as possible.

The following appear to be necessary conditions (in theory) for the development of a suitable *in vitro* method: (1) The activity of the enzyme should be determined in the ambiance of the subject's own plasma without addition of extraneous substrates. (2) Although the available evidence suggests that the use of inhibitors as in the method of *Stokke and Norum* [452] do not affect the enzyme activity, they still should be avoided if at all possible. (3) Radioactive cholesterol should be completely and uniformly incorporated into plasma lipoproteins so that the metabolism of the radioactive cholesterol is comparable to that of the cholesterol native to plasma lipoproteins. (4) The period of incubation for estimating the enzymatic activity should be as short as possible, during which time the activity should be of first order kinetics with respect to time and substrate concentrations.

In vivo/in vitro *Method*

In this method, the plasma FC is labeled *in vivo* either by injecting radioactive precursor such as acetate and mevalonate or by injecting radioactive cholesterol i.v. Usually plasma separated at 4 °C from a blood sample collected (in chilled tubes) 2 h after the injection of labeled precursor is used for incubation and determination of LCAT *in vitro*. The method utilizes the fact that 1–2 h after the injection of radioactive label, the plasma FC is rapidly labeled and the SA of FC in all major lipoprotein classes at this time is identical and compared to it the radioactivity in plasma CE is still rather low [25, 245, 379, 456].

Although this is the ideal method of labeling and determining the LCAT activity *in vitro*, it seems unreasonable to inject radioactivity into humans for the routine determination of LCAT. The method is applicable only in those studies where other investigations are also carried out on cholesterol metabolism using radioisotope techniques.

It is not clear whether the LCAT activities determined *in vitro* reflect the activities of enzyme *in vivo* in both normal and pathological conditions. In this regard, it has been found that LCAT activities determined *in vivo* are identical with those determined *in vitro* in normal subjects [25, 245], but in subjects with hypertriglyceridemia and hypercholesterolemia the LCAT activities as determined *in vivo* were nearly 20% higher than those determined by the *in vivo/in vitro* method [245] in the same subjects.

LCAT Activity during Storage

Plasma samples for the determination of LCAT activities should not be stored at room temperature without adding inhibitors. The samples could be stored at 4 °C; however, the activities should be measured within 5 days after which there is significant reduction. No decrease in activities was found in samples stored at –15 °C up to 4 months [47].

Chapter VII. Catabolism of Cholesterol

The liver is the major organ involved in the catabolism of cholesterol [31,44]. It converts approximately 0.5 g of cholesterol into bile acids in one day [417, 419] and secrets anywhere from 1.0 to 1.5 g of cholesterol in the bile every day [177, 431–433]. Fractions of bile acids and cholesterol secreted into the bile are lost in the feces and the remainder are absorbed from the intestinal tract [30].

Other organs also catabolize significant amounts of cholesterol. Between 0.05 and 0.10 g of cholesterol is lost daily from the skin surface [36, 333] and 0.05 g of cholesterol is removed from plasma and converted into steroid hormones by organs such as adrenal glands, testes, and ovaries [61, 495, 516]. The catabolites of steroid hormones along with trivial amounts of cholesterol are lost in the urine; however, the bulk of cholesterol and its metabolites are lost in the feces. Although the amounts of cholesterol metabolized by extra-hepatic tissues are not trivial, they do not appear to be related to the homeostasis of cholesterol in the plasma. Most of the cholesterol lost from the skin surface is probably synthesized locally by the epidermal cells and the amounts lost do not bear any relationship to the metabolism of plasma lipoproteins [334]. Similarly, the amounts of endogenous cholesterol converted to steroid hormones are probably not influenced by the abnormalities of plasma lipoproteins (although the metabolism of plasma lipoproteins is influenced by the steroid hormones).

In man, liver converts cholesterol to two primary bile acids (fig. 12), i.e. cholic acid and chenodeoxycholic acid. Cholesterol is first transformed into 5β-cholestane-3α,7α,12α-triol, the [27]C bile alcohol. The terminal isopropyl group is then removed from the isooctyl side chain to form the [24]C bile acid; the cholic acid [98, 100]. One pathway for the formation of chenodeoxycholic acid is analogous to the synthesis of cholic acid. The first step is thus the 7α-hydroxylation of cholesterol. The major substrate for 26-hydroxylase is 5β-cholestane-3α,7α-diol. The 7α-hydroxylation is catalyzed by microsomal hydroxylase and soluble factor(s) [100]. Another pathway for synthesis of chenodeoxycholic acid has also been described. It involves an

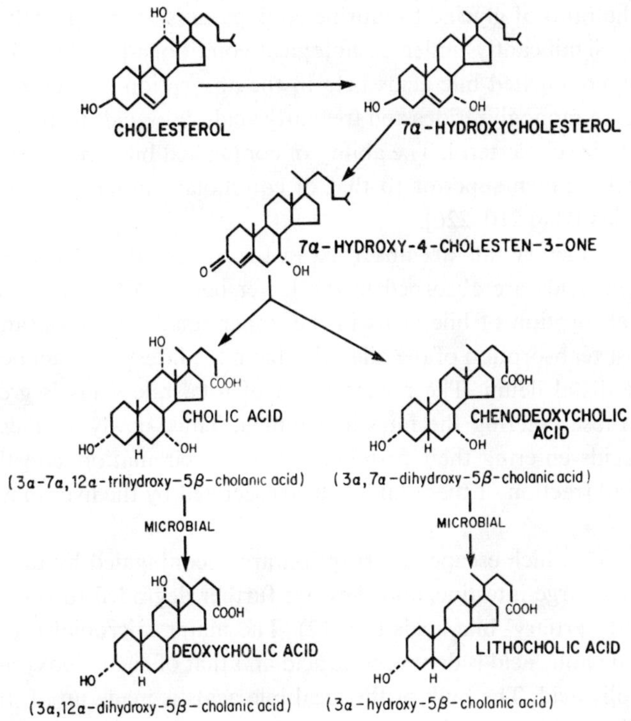

Fig. 12. Hepatic synthesis of primary bile acids (cholic and chenodeoxycholic) from cholesterol and their subsequent degradation to secondary bile acids (deoxycholic and lithocholic) by the intestinal microflora.

initial 26-hydroxylation of cholesterol followed by its oxidation into 3α-hydroxy-5-cholenoic acid, which after many steps is converted to chenodeoxycholic acid. All of these reactions for the second pathway are catalyzed by the mitochondrial fraction fortified with 100,000 g supernatant of the liver cell homogenates [300]. The quantitative significance of these two pathways for synthesis of chenodeoxycholic acid has not yet been established. It appears, however, that 7α-hydroxylation is the rate-limiting reaction in the conversion of cholesterol to all bile acids and it is the site for physiological control of synthesis of bile acids [100, 315].

The two primary bile acids are conjugated in the liver with amino acids, glycine and taurine producing glycocholic, taurocholic, glycochenodeoxycholic, and taurochenodeoxycholic acids [100, 420]. Small fractions of conjugated bile acids may also be present as sulfate esters [279, 343, 345]. In normal bile, the ratio of glycine to taurine conjugates is approximately 3:1, but it can vary significantly under pathological conditions [58, 424]. In the small intestine, conjugated bile acids help in the absorption of dietary fats. In the presence of monoglycerides and free fatty acids, bile acids form micelles which solubilize cholesterol. The ability of conjugated bile acids to solubilize cholesterol is much superior to that of equimolar amounts of unconjugated bile acids [208, 210, 226].

Most of the dietary fats are absorbed in the upper intestines, whereas most of the bile acids are absorbed in the lower ileum. Although there is some passive absorption of bile acids in the upper small intestines (and in the colon), most reabsorption of the bile acids from the intestinal tract occurs actively in the distal ileum. The reabsorption of total bile acids is greater than 98% of those entering the intestinal lumen. Thus, newly synthesized primary bile acids entering their first enterohepatic circulation constitute relatively a small fraction of the total bile acids secreted by the liver in a day [58, 92, 112].

The bile acids which escape reabsorption are deconjugated by the bacterial flora in the large intestine, and they are further degraded to so-called 'secondary' and 'tertiary' bile acids (fig. 12). The major microbial product of deconjugated cholic acid is deoxycholic acid and that of chenodeoxycholic acid is lithocholic acid. The bulk of the fecal bile acids is made up of these 'secondary' bile acids although small amounts of primary bile acids and their other metabolites are also present. In germ-free rats, the feces do not contain secondary or tertiary bile acids [130, 261, 337, 409].

On reabsorption, the deconjugated bile acids are reconjugated in the liver. Recent evidence suggests that most of the reabsorbed lithocholic acid (conjugated with amino acids) is esterified with sulfate; whereas most of the other bile acids are not [91]. This ability of man to esterify lithocholic acid may be a factor in reducing the toxicity of lithocholic acid. Feeding chenodeoxycholic acid to experimental animals causes considerable damage to the liver, whereas such severe toxic reactions to chenodeoxycholic acid administration are not observed in man [149, 447].

The usual methods for the determinations of bile acids in the bile exclude the sulfate esters of lithocholic acid; therefore, biliary bile acids are reported to be present in the following ratios: cholic:chenodeoxycholic:deoxycholic acids 1.1:1.0:0.6 [420]. The total pool of bile acids in man is about 2.5–4.5 g [17, 200, 265, 488]. When the intestinal tract is at rest, most of this pool is concentrated in gallbladder bile; the fresh hepatic bile is low in bile salts [1, 195]. However, after the ingestion of food the gallbladder contracts and forces the bile salts into the intestinal lumen. Most of the biliary bile acids are reabsorbed from the intestines and promptly resecreted by the liver. Therefore, the extent of entero-hepatic circulation of bile acids depends on the number of meals and their composition. It is estimated that the total pool of bile acids undergo 6–10 entero-hepatic circulations, or in other words, more than 15 g of bile acids are secreted in th bile per day [177, 424].

It is often suggested that conversion of cholesterol to bile acids is the major pathway for elimination of cholesterol from the system. Recent and more reliable studies in man, however, indicate that losses of cholesterol from the body pools occur more as fecal cholesterol (or its bacterial derivatives) than as bile acids. Normal subjects on low cholesterol diets excreted $285 \pm$ 169 mg of bile acids a day, whereas the daily losses of fecal cholesterol in the same group were 624 ± 347 mg a day [429]. The fecal excretion of endogenous cholesterol is more susceptible to change in dietary cholesterol than the fecal excretion of bile acids [361, 362]. However, fecal excretion of both cholesterol and bile acids may be significantly affected by the presence or absence of hypertriglyceridemia [236, 325, 431–433].

Methods to Study Synthesis of Bile Acids

For those who are interested in the detailed metabolism of different bile acids and comprehensive discussion of methods, excellent reviews and symposia on the subject are available [211, 213, 294, 315, 424]. For aspects of bile acid metabolism relevant to the turnover of endogenous cholesterol, the available methods can be divided into two broad groups.

(A) Quantitative Methods. (1) Estimation of daily excretion of bile acids in the feces: (a) isotopic methods; (b) chromatographic methods; (c) combination of the two. (2) Isotope dilution method which involves an oral or i.v. dose of radioactive tracer(s) to pulse label one or more bile acids, and the calculation of the turnover rates from the SA decay of bile acid(s).

(B) Qualitative Methods. They give relative rates of hepatic synthesis of bile acids.

Estimation of Daily Excretion of Bile Acids in the Feces

For all practical purposes, fecal excretion represents the only route for the elimination of bile acids from the body. Therefore, in a steady state, the daily fecal excretion of bile acids should equal their daily synthesis of the liver. During the passage of bile acids through the gastrointestinal tract, intestinal microorganisms modify these bile acids extensively, producing a number of different bile acids, thus making specific determinations of each of the bile acids a formidable analytical problem. To circumvent this, *Hellman et al.* [199] introduced a simple isotopic method. The method was based on the assumption that after pulse labeling of plasma cholesterol, the specific activity of biliary bile acids becomes equal to that of plasma cholesterol in 1–7 weeks (depending upon the pool sizes and the turnover rates of cholesterol and bile acids). Once the isotopic equilibrium is reached, the total fecal bile acids can be estimated from the total radioactivity in the fecal extracts containing bile acids and dividing this value by the SA of plasma cholesterol [176]. The theoretical (p. 63) and the analytical (p. 125) details of the method are given elsewhere in the book.

Estimation of fecal bile acids by chemical means involves rather difficult and time-consuming procedures. Some of the problems are: (1) the bile acids may be tightly bound to bacteria or may still be present in conjugated form thus necessitating rigorous and prolonged solvent extraction; (2) feces contain many unknown components which may have chromatographic properties similar to those of fecal bile acids, and (3) when large amounts of free fatty acids are present in the feces, they make chromatographic separation of bile acids difficult. However, recent advances in TLC and GLC and in mass spectrometry have made chemical determinations of various fecal bile acids possible [130, 131, 178].

In 1965, *Grundy et al.* [178] introduced a chemical method for determination of fecal metabolites for endogenous cholesterol which has now become the standard against which other methods are tested. This method involves the use of TLC and GLC and is described in detail on page 125. In a comparative study, the results obtained by isotopic balancem ethods were in good agreement with those obtained by the chromatographic method [175, 247, 248]. The chromatographic balance method gives the synthetic rate for total bile acids and it cannot distinguish between the synthetic rates of cholic and chenodeoxycholic acid. Under steady-state conditions, however, the quantities of fecal deoxycholic and lithocholic acid, and their bacterial metabolites, give some indication of the synthetic rates of the two primary bile acids in the liver. This method eliminates the use of radioactivity and therefore it can be used when the isotopic method is not indicated.

Both isotopic and chromatographic balance methods require complete collection of large pools of feces in order to eliminate the influence of day-to-day variations in fecal flow. This problem, however, can be overcome by feeding non-absorbable fecal markers (p. 133), beginning a few days in advance of fecal collections, thus correcting for the daily variations in the fecal flow [176].

Isotope Dilution Method for Determining the Turnover Rates of Bile Acids
This method was originally introduced by *Lindstedt* [265] and has since been used extensively in man for studies on turnover rates and pool sizes of various bile acids [102, 212, 488, 508]. The method involves i.v. or oral administration of one or more of the labeled bile acids, followed by frequent collection of bile samples for 7–10 days. The assumptions made in this method are: (1) that radioactive tracers mix with the bile acid pools completely before the first sample is taken; (2) that the duodenal aspiration affords a valid sample of the bile acid pool; (3) that the bile acid pool size remains constant during the study; (4) that the oral dose is absorbed as completely as endogenous bile acids, and (5) that there is no hepatic interconversion of the biliary bile acids.

For an accurate estimation of total bile acid synthesis in man, the turnover rates of cholic and chenodeoxycholic acids should be determined simultaneously. This will not give information on the turnover rate or pool size of deoxycholic acid, which can be estimated from the ratios of deoxy to chenodeoxylic acids to the bile, since the absorption of the two is similar [204, 213].

In general, the labeled bile acids are administered i.v. or orally, and samples of duodenal bile are collected every day or every other day for 7–10 days starting from the day after the injection or feeding (hoping that by this time the radioactive bile acids have equilibrated completely with the endogenous pools).

Collection of Duodenal Bile. Under direct examination of fluoroscopic screen, a double lumen tube is passed through the nose or mouth until the 'olive' or mercury bag is approximately 5 cm distal to the ampulla of Vater. A 5% solution of protein hydrolysate infusion or a slow i.v. injection of cholecystokinin-pancreozymin is given to stimulate the contraction of gallbladder, and the tube is clamped for 10 min before aspirating 3–6 ml of bile which is directly mixed with an equal volume of methanol for storage and future analysis [121, 177, 212].

Recently, *Hoffman et al.* [206] have developed a 'non-invasive' procedure for sampling the intestinal content, using a 'sequestering capsule' made up of dialysis tubing containing cholestyramine. During the study period, six capsules are given each day with a meal. The capsules trap conjugated bile acids during their intestinal passage. The capsules are recovered from the feces; the bile acids eluted, isolated chromatographically, and their SA is then determined. The technique appears to yield data identical (but less precise) to those obtained by duodenal sampling [206, 212].

Determination of Pool Sizes and the Turnover Rates of Different Bile Acids
The bile acids are isolated and their SA determined according to the methods described elsewhere (p. 117). The values of SA of bile acids are then plotted against time on a semilogarithmic paper and the half-life as well as the turnover rate constant are calculated for each of the bile acids.

$$Turnover\ rate\ constant,\ K = \frac{0.693}{t\ \frac{1}{2}}.$$

When the exponential slope of the SA decay is extrapolated back to time 0, i.e. to the time when radioactive bile acids are administered, the derived SA at that time represents the dilution of the administered radioactive bile acids in the pool of nonradioactive bile acids present at that time. Thus, the pool size is calculated as follows:

$$Bile\ acid\ pool\ (mg) = \frac{dpm\ injected}{SA_{to}\ (dpm/mg)},$$

Thus, daily synthesis of bile acids $=$ pool size (mg) $\times$ K.

The total pool of bile acids present in the liver, gallbladder, duodenum or the blood can be considered to be parts of the same pool because the decay of SA of bile acids is generally exponential.

The major disadvantage of this method is the requirement of duodenal intubation. Use of sequestering capsules, however, eliminates the need of intubation [206]. Theoretically, it should be possible to determine the SA of serum bile acids and thus avoid duodenal intubation. However, the concentration of serum bile acids is very low, which makes the determinations of radioactivity very difficult, although the concentrations can be determined reasonably well by the use of radioimmunoassay, GLC or enzymatic methods [10, 278, 312, 412].

This method allows estimation of pool sizes as well as synthetic rates of bile acids, each of which has different physiological significance. Changes in one can occur independently of changes in the other.

The values for synthesis (of bile acids) given by this method are ($\simeq 700$

mg/day), considerably higher than those given by chemical or isotopic balance methods ($\simeq$ 300 mg/day). The reasons for this discrepancy in the literature are not apparent. The results were obtained in different laboratories and on different subjects. Most of the earlier studies with isotope dilution methods were done with bile acids labeled generally with tritium; a fraction of which may be lost by isotopic exchange when injected into man [127, 258, 346]. Another reason for the discrepancy may be the presence of impurities. It was found that 15% of the radioactivity present in [2,4-H³]-cholic acid preparation was present in its 3β-OH epimer [346].

When the isotope dilution method was directly compared with chemical balance methods in the same 12 subjects and utilizing the ¹⁴C-labeled bile acids, the results obtained by the methods were comparable. The mean daily total bile acid excretion was 493 mg compared to the mean daily production rate of 487 mg determined by isotope dilution method [487].

However, in a detailed comparative study of the two methods (isotope dilution and chemical balance methods) in 9 subjects, the values for fecal excretion of bile acids were 18–44% lower than those obtained by the isotope dilution method, even when the tracer used was ¹⁴C-bile acids to eliminate the possibility of exchange [455]. This could be due to either an overestimation by the isotope dilution method [303] or underestimation of fecal bile acids by the chemical method. Since the values of fecal bile acids by chemical methods are similar to those obtained by the isotopic balance (not isotope dilution) method [175, 247, 248], it is likely that the isotope dilution method overestimates the pool sizes and thus synthetic rates of bile acids.

Measurement of Hourly Output of Hepatic Secretion of Biliary Lipids

Under certain experimental conditions, it may be necessary to measure the hourly rate of bile acid and cholesterol secretion in bile. Recently, *Grundy and Metzger* [177] developed a method which can evaluate the hourly rates of biliary secretion of all bile lipids. The method employs duodenal intubation with double or triple lumen tubes and infusions of liquid formula containing radioactive or nonradioactive markers. Radioactive cholesterol and radioactive lecithin can be used as markers for cholesterol and phospholipids; β-sitosterol can be used as a single marker for both cholesterol and bile acids.

Method. The subjects are intubated with double or triple lumen tubes the night preceding the study. One tube is 10 cm longer than the other(s). Tubes are tipped with stainless steel olives containing 16 perforations. The distal one is weighted with a mercury bag.

On the day of the study, the proximal olive(s) are placed into the second portion of duodenum near the ampulla of Vater under fluoroscopy. This puts the distal 'olive' just beyond the ligament of Trietz.

Collection of Bile. Liquid formula containing markers is infused at a constant rate so that the total input equals the determined caloric requirement. Constant aspiration of intestinal contents is carried out from the distal (tube 1) and from the proximal sites (tube 2) when triple lumen tubes are used. When the study is carried out for long periods, aspiration rate is reduced to conserve bile acid pool. This can be achieved by filling the tubes 1 and 2 with water at the beginning of each hour.

The aspiration is done in a syringe containing ethanol (5 ml) and the contents are transferred into vials containing methanol (7–5 ml.) After bringing the mixture to a known volume, aliquots are taken for the analysis of cholesterol, bile acids and phospholipids. For analysis, the samples are collected from the distally placed tube and the markers are infused into the proximally placed tube.

Calculations

Cholesterol. The method for the determination of hourly output of biliary cholesterol depends upon the circumstances of the study, i.e. depending on the presence of sterols in the infusion formula and on the type of marker. Cholesterol is extracted from bile as described elsewhere. Radioactivity is counted and depending upon the presence or absence of plant sterols its mass is estimated colorimetrically or by GLC.

When infusion contains cholesterol and the subject under study has previously been given radioactive cholesterol (i.v.), the cholesterol in the infusate should be labeled with a different isotope than the one given i.v. The mass of endogenous cholesterol in the duodenal aspirate is calculated as follows:

Endogenous cholesterol (mg) = radioactivity in endogenous cholesterol (dpm) divided by SA of plasma cholesterol (dpm/mg).

SA of plasma cholesterol is determined simultaneously.

All procedures determine the amount of endogenous cholesterol and exogenous marker in the aspirated sample. Cholesterol output is calculated as follows:

Cholesterol output (mg/h) = Marker input (mg/h) ÷ rate of withdrawal of marker (dpm or mg/h) ÷ rate of withdrawal of endogenous cholesterol (mg/h). (1)

When infusate contains a small amount of exogenous cholesterol, the value for cholesterol withdrawn has to be corrected for the presence of 'exogenous' cholesterol in the infusate. It is assumed that cholesterol is not appreciably absorbed between proximal and distal sites, thus the amounts of exogenous cholesterol withdrawn from the tube 1 is calculated as follows:

Exogenous cholesterol withdrawn (mg/h) = marker withdrawn (mg/h or dpm)
× (exogenous cholesterol input [mg/h] ÷ marker input [dpm or mg/h]).   (2)

The rate of withdrawal of endogenous cholesterol required for equation 1 represents the difference between the total cholesterol and exogenous cholesterol withdrawn.

Bile Acids. Total and/or individual bile acids are extracted from the upper phase, and their mass is determined as described elsewhere. β-Sitosterol is used as a marker and the hourly output is estimated in samples from tube 1 as follows:

Bile acid output (mg/h) = β-sitosterol input (mg/h) ÷ (β-sitosterol withdrawn mg/h ÷ bile acids withdrawn [mg/h]).

Bile acid output is calculated in samples from tube 2 (triple lumen tubes) as follows:

Bile acid output (mg/h) = cholesterol output (mg/h) × (bile acid:cholesterol ratio).

Cholesterol output is obtained in sample from tube 1 as described above and bile acid:cholesterol ratio is obtained in sample from tube 2.

Phospholipids. An equal volume of methanol is added to the aliquot taken for phospholipid analysis. Cholesterol, if radioactive, is removed by extraction with PE and phospholipids are extracted three times with chloroform. Aliquots are then taken for the determination of radioactivity and phosphorus. Radioactive phosphatidyl choline is used as a marker.

Phospholipid output (mg/h) = radioactive phospholipid input (dpm/h) ÷ (radioactive phospholipid withdrawn [dpm/h] ÷ endogenous phospholipid withdrawn [mg/h]).

The following formula gives output of phospholipids when triple lumen tubes are employed:

Phospholipid output (mg/h) = (cholesterol output [mg/h] in sample from tube 1) × (phospholipid:cholesterol ratio in sample from tube 2).

The use of triple lumen tubes eliminates the need for markers for calculation of bile acids and phospholipid outputs; only markers for cholesterol output are necessary.

The results of the hourly output of biliary lipids are valid only in a steady state of *infusion* generally achieved 4–6 h after the start of infusion. This method can give information on the interrelations of biliary lipids and is particularly suitable for the study of acute changes in cholesterol and bile acid excretion, e. g. valuable information on the mobilization of tissue cholesterol can be obtained. If the method is combined with the measurement of fecal excretion of bile acids, a value for absorption of bile acids can be obtained.

Qualitative Methods

These methods are useful in estimating relative rates of synthesis of the bile acids. They are relatively simple, rapid, and can provide useful information about the synthetic rate under different metabolic and dietary conditions.

Estimation of Rate of Bile Acid Synthesis by Measuring $^{14}CO_2$ Production after Administration of [26 or 27-^{14}C]-Cholesterol

During the synthesis of bile acids, the side chain of cholesterol is cleaved leading to the formation of propionyl CoA, 70–90% of which is metabolized to CO_2 and expired [299, 458]. If the side chain of cholesterol is labeled with ^{14}C, the expired $^{14}CO_2$ can be trapped and the radioactivity determined, then the rate of excretion of $^{14}CO_2$ in the breath can be related to the rate of formation of bile acids.

The procedure involves i. v. injection of $\simeq$ 50 μCi of (26 or 27 ^{14}C)-cholesterol and collection of expired air for a known period of time. Before collection, the subject is rested for a few minutes to achieve basal condition. For collection of expired $^{14}CO_2$, a mouthpiece is inserted and the subject is asked to breathe into a Douglas bag for a fixed period. The subject's nose is kept close during this time. The air entering the Douglas bag is passed through a spirometer for the measurement of the volume of air, then over a desiccant to absorb moisture. After collection, an aliquot is pumped into a CO_2-absorbing fluid, and its radioactivity is then determined [314].

Alternatively, sampling of CO_2 can be easily done in a collection system [228] consisting of a mouthpiece made of polyvinyl tubing, one end of which is attached to a vial containing desiccant (for the removal of moisture). The expired air then goes through another polyvinyl tube into a scintillation vial containing 2 ml of 1 M hyamine in methanol and a drop of phenolphthalein solution (1%). Blowing is continued until the alkaline hyamine solution becomes colorless, indicating trapping of exactly 2.0 mmol CO_2. The time required for this is noted. The liquid scintillation vial is removed from the apparatus, 10–15 ml of scintillation fluid is added, and the radioactivity is counted and corrected for quenching. The amount of cholesterol degraded to bile acids per day is estimated as follows:

Bile acids (mg/day) = total $^{14}CO_2$ expired (dpm/day) ÷ SA of plasma cholesterol (dpm/mg).

Since all carbons in the cleaved side chains are not metabolized to CO_2, this method underestimates bile acid synthesis. However, there is a constant relationship between $^{14}CO_2$ formation and cholesterol side chain cleavage, making this method a good indicator of bile acid synthesis [106, 314].

Determination of Hepatic Cholesterol 7α-Hydroxylase Activity

Formation of 7α-hydroxycholesterol is thought to be the first committed step in the biosynthesis of bile acid from cholesterol. The enzyme catalyzing this reaction is mostly found in liver microsomes. A number of different methods are available to determine its activity [39, 97, 225, 301, 407, 484]. In general, the radioactive cholesterol (the substrate) is incubated with suspension of liver microsomes. The 7α-hydroxycholesterol formed is isolated by TLC and from the radioactivity in this fraction, the fraction of radioactive cholesterol converted to 7α-hydroxycholesterol is determined. Recently, *Myant and Mitropoulos* [315] have reviewed the various conditions necessary for the assay of 7α-hydroxylase enzyme.

The method described below was developed by *Nicolau et al.* [331] for the study of the activity of this enzyme in man.

Assay of Cholesterol-7α-Hydroxylase Activity. Liver microsomes are prepared as described earlier (p. 84). The incubation of the microsomal enzyme is carried out in 15-ml culture tubes. The substrate consists of labeled [4^{14}C]-cholesterol (6×10^5 dpm) and unlabeled cholesterol (100 mM) solubilized with 0.75 mg of Cutscum ([isooctyl]-phenoxypolyethylene-ethanol). The substrate (in solution in cyclohexane) and detergent (in acetone solution) are mixed, the organic solvents are evaporated under nitrogen, and the residue is 'solubilized' by vigorous mixing in 0.15 ml of homogenizing medium. The total volume of the assay system is 0.5 ml, consisting of 0.15 ml of an NADPH-generating system with the following composition: potassium phosphate buffer, pH 7.4, 70 mM; MgCl$_2$, 4.5 mM, NADP 1.25 mM (buffered to pH 7.4); glucose-6-phosphate, 2.5 mM (buffered to pH 7.4); glucose-6-phosphate dehydrogenase, 5 enzyme units. The NADPH-generating system is incubated for 5 min at 37 °C before starting the cholesterol 7α-hydroxylase determination. The NADPH-generating system (0.15 ml) is added to the 'solubilized' substrate and the assay is started by adding 0.2 ml of microsomal solution (containing 0.1–3.0 mg of microsomal protein). The mixture is incubated for 20 min at 37 °C in air but taking care to avoid unnecessary exposure to light. A boiled enzyme control is run with each experiment. The reaction is terminated by adding 15–20 volumes of dichloromethane:ethanol 5:1 (v/v) per volume of incubation mixture. Water (2.5 ml) is added; the mixture shaken vigorously in a Vortex mixture for 2 min; and then centrifuged at 2,000 rpm. The organic solvent layer is separated, the extraction repeated once more and the organic phases are combined.

Analysis of 7α-Hydroxycholesterol. Amounts of 7α-hydroxycholesterol may be determined by GLC, by combination of GLC-mass spectrometry or by isotope derivative technique [39, 281, 301, 407]. The isotope derivative technique is simple and could be used routinely. This technique, as developed by *Shefer et al.* [407], is described below and is based on the (nearly) quantitative acetylation of the reaction mixture with labeled acetic anhydride of known SA.

The extract (organic phase) is evaporated under nitrogen at 60 °C. The dried steroid fraction is dissolved in benzene:methanol 4:1 (v/v) and transferred quantitatively in reaction vials. The solvent is evaporated under nitrogen and then evaporated twice after addition of 0.2 ml of benzene:methanol (4:1). The mixture of steroids is then acetylated. For acetylation, 15 μl of a 5% solution of [3H]-acetic anhydride in dry pyridine is added to the steroid mixture. The vials are tightly stoppered and their contents mixed thoroughly. After 6 h at 100 °C, excess [3H]-acetic anhydride and pyridine is removed by repeated addition of benzene:methanol and evaporation under a stream of N$_2$ at 50–60 °C.

The dried, acetylated steroids are dissolved in 50 μl of benzene:methanol 4:1 (v/v) and then applied as a streak (1.5 cm long) to alumina G plates (0.25 mm thickness). Before application to the plates, the plates are activated at 110 °C for 30 min and then transferred onto a hot plate at 40 °C and the acetylated samples are applied to the warm TLC plates. 30–50 μg of unlabeled acetylated sterols are applied to the same streak as carriers. The 7α-(3H,14C)-hydroxycholesterol diacetate formed is separated from its 7β-epimer and from their monoacetylated and unacetylated steroidal contaminants by TLC with peroxide-free ether:hexane 1:1 (v/v) as the solvent system. The sterols are made visible by spraying lightly with 3.5% phosphomolybdic acid in isopropanol. The pertinent bands are removed and transferred into a scintillation vial containing 0.3 ml of water and 14 ml of scintillation solution (consisting of 5 g 2,5-diphenyloxazole and 100 g of naphthalene per liter of dioxane). After counting, suitable corrections are made for background, crossover, and efficiencies of the ^{3}H and ^{14}C labels. Losses during extraction, acetylation, and other handling procedures can be corrected by comparing the ^{14}C counts found in the acetylated steroids with the initial counts added or by using a known amount (50 nmol) of unlabeled 7β-hydroxycholesterol, added after the incubation, as internal standard.

The results are corrected for the non-enzymatic oxidation of cholesterol by subtracting values obtained for the boiled enzyme (control). The net amount of 7α-hydroxycholesterol synthesized during incubation is calculated as follows:

7α-Hydroxycholesterol formed (μmol) = total ^{3}H (dpm) in 7α-hydroxycholesterol diacetate ÷ SA of [^{3}H]-acetic anhydride (dpm/μmol).

The solvent used to dissolve the exogenous substrate (i.e. acetone or detergent) affects the determination of the 7α-hydroxylase activity. The activity is considerably lower when acetone is used than when a detergent is used to dissolve the exogenous substrate [23, 40].

Recently, *Van Cantfort et al.* [484] and *Johnson et al.* [225] described a simple method based on the release of ^{3}H from [7α-^{3}H]-cholesterol following its enzymatic conversion to 7α-hydroxycholesterol. Incubation of liver microsomes with [7α-^{3}H]-cholesterol or [7α,7β-^{3}H]-cholesterol releases the labeled hydrogen in the 7α position as ^{3}H$_2$O which, after counting, allows for the determination of fraction of exogenous cholesterol converted to 7α-hydroxycholesterol.

The method in brief involves the incubation of liver microsomes using [7α-^{3}H]-cholesterol or [7α, 7β-^{3}H]-cholesterol as the exogenous substrate. Preparation of microsomes and incubation procedure is same as described earlier. At the end of the incubation period, the reaction is terminated by adding 12 volumes of dry methylene chloride. The tube is centrifuged at 1,500 rpm to separate the aqueous phase. An aliquot of the aqueous phase (top layer) is placed in the limb of a Rittenberg tube; the aliquot is purified and sublimated into ice. Aliquots of the thawed ice are then assayed for tritium content and then related to the total water content [225].

The method has been tested under different metabolic conditions and has been found to accurately reflect the enzymic activity. The method is simple, rapid, and is independent of further metabolism of the first enzymatic product, the 7α-hydroxycholesterol [484].

Extraction, Purification, Separation, and Quantitation of Bile Acids

A number of different methods are available for the extraction, purification, separation, and estimation of conjugated and free bile acids from biological samples. The choice of the method therefore will depend upon the purpose of the experiment. The procedure is much simpler if only the total amounts of the conjugated or free bile acids are required than if the concentrations of the individual bile acids are needed. The individual bile acids need to be separated by TLC after their extraction and hydrolysis. Separation and quantitation could also be done by GLC without TLC.

Extraction of Bile Acids from Bile and Duodenal Secretion

Bile or duodenal juice is centrifuged at 3,000 rpm for 10 min to sediment solids and other suspended particles. A measured volume of bile or the duodenal juice (1–2 ml) is added to 20 times the volume of chloroform: methanol (2:1 v/v). The mixture is heated in a water bath at 80 °C for 10 min to precipitate proteins. The solution is then filtered through glass wool or Whatman No. 1 filter paper into a graduated cylinder, and the protein residue on the filter is washed with the same solvent. Distilled water 0.2 times the volume of the solvents is added and the mixture is shaken and allowed to separate into two phases. The top layer containing conjugated bile acids is removed as completely as possible by siphoning; additional distilled water equal to 0.2 times the volume of the lower phase is added and mixed again. The top aqueous phase is removed and pooled with the first layer. The combined top aqueous layers are evaporated to dryness under reduced pressure at 75 °C and the residue dissolved in a known volume of methanol:water (85:15). The bottom layer can then be used for estimation of cholesterol and phospholipids [27, 410].

Conjugated Bile Acids

To obtain conjugated bile acids, the bile or duodenal juice could also be extracted with 4 volumes of methanol:acetone (1:1 v/v) [134, 507] or with 5 volumes of 95% ethanol or by 9 volumes of chloroform:methanol (9:1) [123, 260]. Before extraction, the bile acid containing aqueous 'micellar phase' could be physically separated by centrifuging at 100,000 g for 16–18 h. On centrifugation, the sample separates into three phases: a Pellet containing solids; an aqueous phase containing bile acids, and an oily layer containing other lipids. The whole aqueous phase is carefully removed by piercing the centrifuge tube with a needle and withdrawing the fluid into a syringe. The 'micellar phase' could be used directly for estimation of bile acids or could be extracted before quantitation [21, 341].

Free Bile Acids

For a detailed study of the bile acid composition, it is usually necessary to hydrolyze the conjugated bile acids since conjugated chenodeoxycholic acid and deoxycholic acid cannot be separated easily. Conversion to free bile acids facilitates their extraction into organic solvents and subsequent separation and quantitation. Hydrolysis could be accomplished either by alkaline hydrolysis or by enzymatic cleavage.

Alkaline Hydrolysis

The conditions described for hydrolysis vary considerably. Extensive destruction of common bile acids may occur during this process. Use of glass tubes may result in losses due to adsorption especially if microgram amounts of bile acids are involved. Losses appear to be relatively small if borosilicate tubes are used and milligram quantities of bile acids are involved. Teflon tubes in a pressure cooker or Parr bombs in a routine oven could also be used [213].

The bile or the duodenal juice extract is evaporated to dryness and the residue is dissolved in an appropriate quantity of 2 N sodium hydroxide (5–15 ml); the mixture is saponified at 2 atmospheres (15 psi) for 3 h in a pressure cooker [178]. Alternatively, they can be rapidly hydrolyzed with ethylene glycol-KOH at 150 °C [131]; however, some losses do occur which could be monitored with the use of internal standards (usually radiolabeled conjugated bile acids). If the bile or the duodenal juice is hydrolyzed directly, concomitant hydrolysis and interference from other lipids (fatty acids) may necessitate purification of bile acids by TLC [213].

Enzymatic Cleavage

The hydrolysis of conjugated bile acids can be conveniently carried out by an enzyme, N-cholylglycine hydrolase (EC 3.5), which specifically hydrolyses naturally occurring bile acid conjugates [317, 318]. The enzyme may be prepared from *Clostridia* or obtained commercially. If kept frozen, the prepared enzyme appears to be stable for 1 year.

Bile or the duodenal juice extract (0.1–0.2 ml) is added to 10 ml of 0.1 M acetate buffer (pH 5.6) containing 7.8 mg of 2-mercaptoethanol and 37 mg of disodium EDTA. To this is added 0.1–2.0 ml of the enzyme (SA not less than 100 μmol/mg protein) and the mixture is incubated at 37 °C for 25–30 min. The incubation mixture is then cooled to room temperature.

Extraction of Free Bile Acids

After alkaline or the enzymatic hydrolysis of bile acid conjugates, the mixture is cooled, some distilled water is added (5–10 ml), and then acidified to pH 1–2 with addition of 6 N HCL. Free bile acids are extracted three times with 25 volumes of ethyl ether or chloroform:methanol (2:1) [178, 213, 410]. Combined extracts are taken to dryness under a stream of nitrogen and the bile acids dissolved in 0.5 ml of ethanol for TLC.

For quantitative recovery of bile acids from their taurine and glycine derivatives, enzymatic hydrolysis is to be preferred over alkaline hydrolysis [382]. Enzymatic hydrolysis, however, may not hydrolyze sulfated bile acids. It was shown recently that lithochoolic acid is present in bile as the sulfate and that the conventional alkaline hydrolysis procedure destroys bile acid sulfates. A solvolysis step preceding alkaline hydrolysis was therefore proposed [345]. However, *Hofmann* and his associates [483] found that the proportion of lithocholate in biliary bile acids was similar whether or not solvolysis procedure preceded deconjugation by alkaline hydrolysis. These workers (based on their extensive experience) have developed an improved method for complete recovery of bile acids in bile.

The method involves addition of 9 volumes of distilled isopropanol to 1 volume of bile. After centrifuging, an aliquot of the supernatant is transferred to Paar bomb. A suitable internal standard is added and mild alkaline hydrolysis in 8 ml of 1.7 N NaOH-methanol (3:1) is carried out for 4 h at 115 °C. The saponification mixture is transferred to a tube in an ice bath and acidified to pH 1 with 5 ml concentrated HCl (12.5 M). Three volumes of ether is added and the mixture is shaken thoroughly and the incubated for 20 min. This procedure completely hydrolyses bile acid conjugates and sulfates without destruction of bile acid structure. The free bile acids are then completely extracted with two additional extractions with 3 volumes of ether. The ether extracts are then evaporated to dryness and bile acids dissolved in a known volume of an appropriate solvent.

Separation of Bile Acids

An aliquot of the bile extract (containing either conjugated or free bile acids) is applied to silica gel G plates. A solution of standards containing known conjugated or free bile acids should also be applied alongside the plate. Application can be done as a streak (for large quantities) or as spots (for μg amounts). When samples are applied, the plates must not be heated as some of the bile acids are adsorbed to the silica gel and they do not move in the chromatographic system. It is a good practice to clean the silica gel plates by prerunning the plates in chloroform:methanol:water (85:35:5 v/v). The plates should be dried and activated before use (120°C for 1 h).

Conjugated and free dihydroxycholanic acids are generally difficult to separate by TLC. A number of solvent systems have been suggested for their separation, most of which will separate them from cholic and lithocholic acids as well. Deoxycholic acid can be separated from chenodeoxycholic acid more easily if they are first converted to methyl esters. Methyl esters can be prepared by treating the methanolic extract with excess ethereal diazomethane in a vial [216]. After 15 min, the volatile components are removed under nitrogen and the procedure is repeated to ensure complete conversion to methyl esters. The interfering lipids (phospholipids, cholesterol, fatty acids, etc.) are generally well resolved in most of these solvent systems. In most of the systems, phospholipids generally stay at the point of application while cholesterol, fatty acids and other neutral lipids move to the top of the plate. In some cases, it may be necessary to first develop the plate in a one solvent system for the removal of neutral lipids (which may interfere with the separation and quantitation of bile acids) and then in a second solvent system for separation of bile acids. Some of the solvent systems and their volume used for the separation of conjugated and free bile acids or their methyl esters by TLC are given below.

For conjugated bile acids: (1) isoamylacetate:propionic acid:propanol: water (4:3:2:1) [207]; (2) isoamylacetate:propionic acid:propanol:water (6:6:4:3) [209]; (3) isooctane:diisopropyl ether:glacial acetic acid:n-butanol:isopropanol:water (10:5:5:3:6:1) [218]; (4) n-butanol:acetic acid: water (10:1:1) [150]; (5) toluene:acetic acid:water (10:10:1) [274].

For free bile acids or their methyl esters: (1) isooctane:ethylene chloride acetic acid (2:1:1) [174, 189]; (2) Isooctane:ethylacetate:acetic acid (5:5:1): [129]; (3) isooctane:ethylacetate:acetic acid:n-butanol (10:5:1.5:1.5) [460]; (4) isooctane:diisopropylether:acetic acid:n-butanol:water (10:5:5:3:1) [218]; (5) isooctane:isopropanol:acetic acid (120:40:1) [178]; (6) isoamylacetate : n-propanol : diisopropylether : carbontetrachloride: benzene: acetic acid (8:5:6:4:2:1) [207; (7) PE:isopropylether:acetic acid (2:1:1) [410]; (8) chloroform:acetone:methanol:acetic acid (70:20:5:1) [209].

Before development of the plates, the solvent system is allowed to equilibrate for 1 h in the chamber (lined with filter paper). The plate is developed, removed, and dried at room temperature before visualization of the separated bile acid bands.

Detection of Bile Acids on Thin Layer Plates

A number of different methods and color reagents (table I) are available for the detection of the bile acids after their separation by TLC. The choice of the spray agent depends upon whether one wants to qualitatively identify the bile acids or whether one is interested in their quantitation after identification. Most of the spray reagents are destructive to the bile acid molecule and so their use precludes further quantification. They are useful for photographic presentation. They could, however, be used for detection if care is taken to protect the area of the plate from which the bile acids are to be quantitated. This could be done by tightly wrapping the area of the plate in a saran wrap and spraying only that portion containing the standard bile acids applied to facilitate identification.

Alternatively, nondestructive methods could be used to visualize the bile acids on plates. These methods do not help in identification of the bile acids unless the standards are applied individually. The bile acids may be detected by spraying the plate with distilled water. The bile acids appear as white dry spots on a gray wet background. The developed chromatograms can also be exposed briefly to iodine vapor. Iodine sublimates easily without heating and does not interfere with subsequent quantitative determination. The plate could also be sprayed with 0.05% pyrene in PE (BP 60–80 °C), and the bile acids visualized under UV light (350 nm). Pyrene can then be removed to the top of the plate using chloroform:PE (9:1). Free or conjugated bile acids do not move in this system [123].

After visualization, the outline of the areas occupied by the bile acids are marked by a needle and the silica gel scraped off quantitatively for elution. Alternatively, they can be processed further without elution. Silica gel can also be scraped off the plate and collected in tubes using vacuum aspirators.

Quantitation of Bile Acids

A number of different methods are available for estimating conjugated and free bile acids. They may be estimated by: (1) colorimetric; (2) fluorometric, and (3) enzymatic methods. Free bile acids may also be estimated by GLC methods.

Colorimetric Method
The Sulphuric Acid Chromogen
The spots are scraped directly into conical centrifuge tubes (bile acid eluates after evaporating the solvent could also be used). 4 ml of 65% sulphuric acid is added and mixed thoroughly using a Vortex mixture and allowed to stand for 15 min at room temperature. After centrifugation for 10 min at 3,000 rpm, the supernatant is decanted into cuvets and optical density at 320 nm is determined. A blank sample of the adsorbent is treated similarly.

Since conjugated chenodeoxycholic acid and deoxycholic acids cannot be separated on TLC, they are estimated together. Their individual quantities, however, can be estimated semiquantitatively from the difference in their absorption maxima. After adding 65% sulphuric acid and mixing, the tubes are heated at 60 °C for 60 min. When this is done, the conjugated deoxycholic acid has an absorption maxima at 389 nm, whereas conjugated chenodeoxycholic acid has a maximum at 305 nm [213, 421].

The Pettenkofer Chromogen
To the silica gel in centrifuge tubes (or eluates of bile acids) 5 ml of 70% sulphuric acid is added and left after mixing at 42 ± 2 °C for 10 min. 1 ml of 0.25% solution of furfural is then added and the contents are thoroughly mixed and allowed to stand for 1 h. The tubes are then centrifuged for 25 min at 3,500 rpm (not necessary if the eluates of bile acids are used), the supernatant removed into cuvets and the color read at 510 nm 90 min after addition of furfural. The amounts of free bile acid or conjugated bile acid is estimated by comparison with a calibration graph obtained from known amounts of the appropriate bile acids [65, 123].

The Pettenkofer reaction is sensitive for cholic, chenodeoxycholic, deoxycholic, and hyodeoxycholic acid and their taurine and glycine conjugates, but is of no use in the estimation of muricholic or the monohydroxylated (lithocholic) acids [123].

It was found that peroxides and certain metal ions influence the chromogen formation, e.g. presence of iron has been shown to inhibit the Petten-kofer reaction [123]. It is therefore necessary that the silica gel is cleaned thoroughly before use, similarly the solvents used for extracts and chromatography should be peroxide-free, and should be tested before use.

Salicylaldehyde Chromogen

This procedure is used for quantitation of conjugated deoxycholic acid in presence of conjugated chenodeoxycholic acid. The procedure utilizes the fact that the color, developed on adding salicylaldehyde is specific for deoxycholic acid [468]. Its taurine and glycine conjugates have identical absorption curves with a peak at 700 nm, while conjugates of chenodeoxycholic acid have a very low absorbance at this wavelength (amounting to about 3% of the extinction for the corresponding deoxycholic conjugates for the same amount of the two substances).

Silica gel containing the bile acids (TDC+TCDC or GDC + GCD) is transferred into test tubes and 600 μl of salicylaldehyde reagent (0.1 ml salicylaldehyde thoroughly mixed with 3.4 ml of 65% sulphuric acid) is added and mixed throroughly. Tubes are heated at 40 °C for 15 min and then 4 ml of glacial acetic acid is added and mixed again for 10 sec. The mixture is centrifuged at 3,000 rpm for 5 min.

The supernatant is transferred into a cuvet and color is read at 700nm exactly 15 min after addition of the acetic acid, together with a blank consisting of an equivalent area of silica gel treated similarly as the unknown. The quantitation is done using standard curves. The color, after addition of acetic acid, is not stable; therefore, the time between addition of acetic acid and reading is important and should remain constant [71].

Fluorometric Method

The silica gel corresponding to sample spots is scraped off the plate and placed in a centrifuge tube. Silica gel spots containing no samples are also taken as blanks. Fluorescence is developed by adding 5 ml of 96.5% of sulphuric acid. After addition of sulphuric acid, the tubes are thoroughly mixed and heated in a water bath at 65 °C for exactly 60 min. The tubes are then cooled and centrifuged at 3,000 rpm for 10 min to sediment silica gel. The wavelength for excitation is 436 nm and the fluorescence is measured at 510 nm. Standard curves of individual bile acids are prepared for the quantitation of the bile acids [21, 147, 260].

It must be pointed out that the fluorescence is influenced by the presence of a variety of substances. The thin-layer plates must be thoroughly dry because alcohol components of the solvent system fluoresce strongly in the region of measurement, following treatment with concentrated sulphuric acid. Also, since the wavelengths of exciting and emitted light are of great importance, it is necessary to test and standardize any fluorescence method with the particular fluorometer used [21].

Enzymatic Method

Iwata and Yamasaki [224] described a method for quantitative determination of bile acids by the use of 3α-hydroxysteroid dehydrogenase (3α-HSDH). The enzyme which is produced by *Pseudomonas testosteroni* specifically oxidizes the 3α-hydroxyl group in the presence of NAD, resulting in the conversion of the 3α-OH group to the 3-keto group and the stoichiometric reduction of NAD to NADH. The reduced NADH is measured spectrophotometrically at 340 nm, or alternatively the sensitivity of the method could be increased by fluorometric detection of NADH using an excitation wavelength at 365 nm and an emission wavelength at 472 nm. The addition of hydrazine as a ketone-trapping agent forces the reaction essentially to completion in 30 min [71].

It has been found that precipitation of proteins as well as extraction of lipids from bile or duodenal aspirates is unnecessary for the determination of the total bile acid concentration. Similarly, elution of bile acids from silica gel is not necessary. At low concentrations of bile acids, free fatty acids, however, strongly inhibit the reaction [134]. The method has also been used for the estimation of fecal bile acids [408, 492].

Recently, another enzyme, 7α-hydroxysteroid dehydrogenase (7α-HSDH), has been isolated from *Escherichia coli* strain 23 which specifically oxidizes the 7α-hydroxyl group. The use of 3α-HSDH in parallel with 7α-HSDH which specifically estimates chenodeoxycholic acid (3α,7α) in presence of deoxycholic acid (3α,12α) permits one to measure all the major 3α-hydroxy bile acids present in the biological material after their separation by TLC [273, 275].

Enzymatic methods for determination of bile acids therefore represents a major advance over colorimetric and other procedures with respect to specificity, sensitivity, and simplicity.

Enzymatic Assay

No standard assay system has been described for the estimation of bile acids by the enzymatic procedure. The assay procedure given below was described by *MacDonald et al.* [274]. Complete oxidations by both 3α-

HSDH and 7α-HSDH can be performed simultaneously in separate tubes. Silica gel spots containing bile acids can be taken as such in which case samples should be dissolved in 0.5 ml of methanol:water (3:1) or the samples can be first eluted with methanol, evaporated to dryness, and then reconstituted in 0.2 ml of methanol:water (3:1).

The assay system consists of NAD ($1.7 \times 10^{-3}M$), glycine -NaOH buffer (0.05 M, pH 9.5), and the bile acids sample (4–24 μm). The reaction is initiated by adding 0.1 ml of freshly prepared solution of 3α-HSDH (1 mg/ml) to all samples including blanks, and 0.1 ml of freshly prepared 7α-HSDH (3–4 mg/ml) to the tubes containing chenodeoxycholic acid (total reaction volume 3 ml, pH 9.2). The mixture is incubated at room temperature for 40 min, mixing at every 5 min for a period of 10 sec. After incubation, the absorbance is read at 340 nm in cuvets of 1-cm light path. If silica gel is present, then the silica gel is separated by centrifugation at 3,000 rpm for 10 min before measuring the absorbance.

As the enzymes specifically oxidizes the 3α-OH or 7α-OH group, the amount of NADH formed is proportional to the amount of bile acid oxidized. Therefore, concentration of bile acid in the unknown sample expressed as μmol can be calculated from the formula $\dfrac{\Delta E \times 3}{6.2}$ μmol, where ΔE is the extinction of the unknown sample, 6.2 is the μmolar extinction coefficient of NADH at 340 nm, and 3 is the total volume of the reaction mixture.

The bile acid oxidized by 7α-HSDH represents the concentration of chenoxydeoxycholic acid while that oxidized by 3α-HSDH represents the total concentration of chenodeoxycholic and deoxycholic acid in samples containing both acids. The concentration of deoxycholic acid is thus given by formula:

(GCDC + GDC)3α-oxid−(GCDC)7α-oxid = (GDC)

Similarly,

(TCDC + TDC)3α-oxid−(TCDC)7α-oxid = (TDC).

Thus, using the combined enzymatic method, concentration of each conjugated or free bile acids can be determined individually after separation by TLC.

GLC Methods

Bile acids may also be determined by GLC with or without prior separation by TLC [130, 178, 251, 421]. Conjugated bile acids cannot be analyzed by GLC and therefore must be first hydrolyzed. The sample containing free bile acids is first methylated using excess etherial diazomethane or 5% HCl gas in super dry methanol. Trimethyl silyl ethers or trifluoroacetates are then prepared. The reagents are evaporated and the residue dissolved in a suitable volume of ethyl acetate and an accurately measured aliquot (between 2 and 5 μl) is injected into a gas chromatograph. A number of different columns have been used. Most commonly used columns are 6-feet silanized glass columns filled with 3% QF1, or 2% OV210 (for trifluoroacetates) or 3% HiEFF8BP (for trimethyl-silyl ethers) on acid washed gas chrom q, 100–120 mesh. A hydrogen detector is used and the general conditions are as follows: column 220 °C; flash heater 240 °C; detector 250 °C, and carrier gas helium 50–50 ml/min.

Cholestane, nordeoxycholic acid or hyocholic acid may be used as an internal standard [131, 178, 454]. The latter two can be added at the initial stage and can be followed through the entire procedure including GLC measurement of individual bile acid methyl esters after their separation by TLC.

Quantities of bile acids in the sample are determined by comparison of peak areas with those of known amounts of reference compounds in a range where a linear detector response is obtained.

The details of this method for the estimation of fecal bile acids are given on page 131.

Determination of SA of Bile Acids

To determine SA, the bile acid must be isolated. Its radioactivity is then determined by liquid scintillation spectrometry and the mass is determined by one of the above methods.

The most commonly used scintillation fluid for counting radioactivity consists of 4 g PPO (2,5-diphenyloxazole) and 0.05 g POPOP (1,4 *bis*[4-methyl-5-phenyloxazolyl]-benzene), dissolved in 1 liter of toluene. Conjugated or free bile acids are usually dissolved in 0.5 ml ethanol before the addition of scintillation fluid. Silica gel spots containing the radioactive bile acids could also be counted. 0.5 ml of ethanol is added to dissolve the bile acids. Counting can be done using either glass or polyethylene vials. Quenching should be corrected by the use of internal or external standardization method.

Chapter VIII. Cholesterol Balance Method
for the Study of Cholesterol Metabolism in Man

Cholesterol balance is perhaps the most important concept developed for reliable studies on different parameters of cholesterol metabolism in man [178, 296]. The method is based on the fact that losses of endogenous cholesterol and its metabolites occur predominantly in the feces. Although there are additional losses of endogenous cholesterol from the skin surface (as cholesterol) and in the urine (as metabolites of steroid hormones synthesized from cholesterol), they are not influenced by abnormalities of cholesterol metabolism seen in hyperlipoproteinemias [36, 333]. On a cholesterol-free diet, the amounts of cholesterol and its metabolites lost in the feces represent the net synthesis of cholesterol in the body (however, for greater accuracy, one may add to it the amounts lost through the skin surface and in the urine). The fecal products of cholesterol can be measured either by isotopic methods [176, 199] or by chromatographic methods [178, 296]. The combined use of isotopic and chromatographic methods can give additional information which is not available from any of the two methods when used alone, i.e. absorption of dietary cholesterol [175, 176].

Only the practical details of the method will be given in this section. The theoretical basis underlying the approach in discussed earlier on page 46.

Steady-State Conditions

A metabolic steady state is a necessary prerequisite of the cholesterol balance methods. Not only the amounts and the composition of the dietary intake should remain constant from day to day, the subject should also be in equilibrium with the environment so that there are no significant changes either in body weight or in plasma cholesterol levels (or for that matter, any other pools of cholesterol present in the body). The steady state also implies a constant amount of fecal excretion of neutral and acidic metabolites of endogenous cholesterol.

Diet

Diet is one of the most important factors in maintaining the metabolic steady state. Both liquid formula [89, 179] and solid food diets [215, 237] have been used in cholesterol balance studies. Liquid formula diets of constant composition can be prepared in large batches, and their intake from meal to meal and day to day can be kept constant rather easily [7]. Moreover, the proportions of the dietary proteins, fats, and carbohydrates, as well as the amounts of dietary cholesterol and plant sterols, can be manipulated and monitored more easily than is the case with solid food diets. When it is necessary to feed a constant amount of radioactive cholesterol with the same SA from meal to meal and from day to day, a liquid formula diet is the obvious solution since it is extremely difficult to devise a solid foot diet to achieve this end.

However, the liquid formula diets also have some disadvantages. They do not represent the form of diet that we habitually consume. Although the proportions and the amounts of proteins, carbohydrates, and fats, as well as the content of cholesterol and plant sterols may be made comparable to those in a diet habitually consumed by any given subject, the liquid formula diets do not represent the normal food in all of its aspects. For example, the liquid formula diets are generally devoid of roughage, and since they fail to add significant bulk to the intestinal contents, it may be associated with decreased intestinal motility. It has also been shown that presence of unabsorbed fiber in the diet is associated with increased excretion of bile acids in experimental animals [242]. It is therefore conceivable that the fecal excretion of bile acids on liquid formula diets may be somewhat less than that on solid foot diets. The possibility of liquid formula diet influencing the intestinal microflora and their metabolic consequences also needs to be considered. *Grundy et al.* [179] observed considerable amounts of unexplained losses of neutral sterols (cholesterol as well as plant sterols) in the intestinal tract of the subjects on liquid formula diets. Such losses, however, are generally not seen in subjects consuming solid food diets [237, 248]. It is possible that the differences in the two may well be related to the intestinal microflora in the two groups of subjects. *Denbesten et al.* [110] demonstrated that significant losses of neutral steroids occurred when a subject was given liquid formula diet, but not when the same subject was fed solid food diet of the same composition. They also demonstrated that the addition of cellulose to the liquid formula diet prevented the (unexplained) losses observed when the subject was on a liquid formula diet.

It is therefore obvious, that the use of solid food diets may be more appropriate from the standpoint of normal eating habits of the general population. However, the consumption of solid food diets is more difficult to manipulate and to keep constant from day to day. Nonetheless, a reasonably steady state of cholesterol metabolism can be achieved in subjects on solid food diets even on an outpatient basis. Whenever possible, the patients should be admitted to the metabolic ward in a hospital. Unlike the crystalline cholesterol suspended in liquid formula diets, the cholesterol and the plant sterols in the solid food diets are integral components of the consumed items. One is, therefore, not concerned with the physical state or the dispersion of cholesterol when using solid food diets. On the other hand, it is extremely difficult to design a solid food diet containing constant amounts of cholesterol with a constant SA, and to ensure uniformity of all meals within a day and on a day-to-day basis. For most purposes, however, it is possible to prepare and freeze individual meals of solid food diets which are reasonably constant in composition. The portions are taken from a single pool of a given item of food. This is particularly important in the case of meat, since even in the same cut of meat from different animals the relative amounts of fat and cholesterol may vary with age and other characteristics of the animal. Items such as slices of bread, skim milk, butter or margarine, cheese, and cereals can be accurately weighed and dispensed without the necessity of having to freeze them. Similarly, the fruits and vegetables can also be accurately weighed and given to the subjects on a day-to-day basis.

It is necessary that each subject be allowed to equilibrate with experimental diets before the studies are undertaken. In general, the more different the experimental diet from the habitual intake of the subject, the longer should be the period of equilibration. The subject is asked to keep a detailed diary of his daily intake over a period of 1 week which is analyzed by a dietician to determine the composition of the diet and calories consumed by the subject. The dietician then designs an experimental diet based on this information so that the experimental diet for each individual resembles his or her habitual intake as closely as possible, and a period of 1 week may be considered to be more or less adequate for equilibration. During this week, the caloric intake is adjusted to maintain the body weight and the patient is also allowed to modify the diet to suit individual preferences. Depending on one's objective, all subjects in the same study may be given the same diet, differing perhaps only with respect to the number of calories, in which case longer periods of equilibration on experimental diets will be necessary.

Although some plant sterols are integral parts of the experimental solid food diets, it is advisable to supplement their intake by adding about 100 mg of β-sitosterol to each meal. By adding such relatively small amounts of plant sterols and keeping these amounts constant from day to day, the effects of variation of sterol content in daily food can be minimized. Such amounts of plant sterols, however, do not significantly influence the absorption of cholesterol, while providing an excellent basis for monitoring the dietary intake.

Selection of Subjects

Cholesterol balance studies are time-consuming and expensive for the investigators and they also put substantial demands on the subjects. It is therefore important that the subject be selected with particular care. The objectives and the rationale of the study should be explained in detail to the subjects and they should understand that they will be facing the restrictions of an experimental diet, discomfort of repeated blood samples, and the monotony of prolonged hospital stay under close supervision. Only those subjects should be enrolled into the study who understand the protocol and who are considered disciplined enough to comply with it. It is also important to make a note of medications needed for unrelated disorders.

Facilities

Ideally, the balance studies should be done in a metabolic ward of the hospital. Facilities in a metabolic ward generally include competent nurses and nutritionists to ensure proper intake as well as quantitative collections. However, it is also possible to study reliable candidates on an outpatient basis, so long as there are means to adequately control and dispense the diets. The subjects may be called to the hospital for all their meals under close supervision. We have also been able to freeze portions for individual meals which were consumed by the subjects at home. Fecal recoveries of dietary β-sitosterol were used to monitor the intake. The results obtained in patients studied on an outpatient basis were no different from those studied in the metabolic ward. It should be appreciated that such studies cannot be done without complete cooperation of the patient (and spouse) and close supervision of a nutritionist, even if the patients are in a metabolic ward.

Clinical Methods in Study of Cholesterol Metabolism

122

Labeling of Plasma Cholesterol

For estimation of fecal sterols by isotopic methods, the plasma cholesterol has to be labeled with radioactive (^{14}C or ^3H) cholesterol at least 4–6
weeks before beginning the metabolic investigations. The studies should not
be started until the decline in the SA of plasma cholesterol becomes exponential.

Labeling of plasma cholesterol can be achieved by any one of the methods discussed on page 39. The i.v. injections of an alcoholic suspension of
radioactive cholesterol in physiological saline is about the simplest procedure
and is described below.

The required amount (50 μCi of 4-^{14}C-cholesterol or 100 μCi of 1-2-
^3H-cholesterol) is taken up in 1 ml of ethanol and dispersed in 150 ml of
physiological saline for administration as an i.v. drip. Alternatively, the i.v.
infusion of physiological saline is first started and the radioactive cholesterol
is injected slowly taking at least 5 min and then rinsing the syringe repeatedly.
To facilitate the injection of radioactive cholesterol, the physiological saline
is infused through a surgical veno-pack which has a side arm for injection.
Approximately 50 ml of the physiological saline is allowed to flow through
the needle and into the vein after completing the injection so as to flush the
radioactivity from the sides of the tubing. After completing the injection, the
needle, syringe and the tubing (which came in contact with the radioactivity)
are washed with the methanol and the radioactivity determined. This is then
subtracted from the amount of radioactivity initially taken up for i.v. injections to determine the precise amount of radioactivity injected into the body.

Beginning a week before the start of the experimental diet, the subject
is given chromic oxide (100 mg t.i.d. with meals) which is continued until the
end of the study. It takes anywhere from 1–2 weeks for the chromic oxide to
achieve balance, i.e. the daily excretion of chromic oxide equals the daily
intake. Some individuals fail to obtain balance even after a period of weeks,
and such subjects are not considered reliable for cholesterol balance studies
[105]. However, *Kottke and Subbiah* [237] suggest that even if the subject is
apparently excreting only 30% of the ingested chromic oxide, the data can
be adequately corrected and satisfactory results obtained.

After the SA of plasma cholesterol begins to decline exponentially, the
subject is given the experimental diet. During the first 7–10 days, the caloric
intake is adjusted to ensure maintenance of body weight. The patient is also
allowed a certain degree of adjustments to ensure his compliance. After this
period of adjustment and equilibration, the exact 'transit time' is determined
for each subject. The subject is given a single capsule containing $\simeq$ 300 mg

of carmine red, and the time taken for the bulk of the dye to appear in the feces is noted.

Collection of Stools

Next to the diet, the most important aspect of the balance studies is the quantitative collection of feces. *Ahrens* and his associates [5–7], the developers of the cholesterol balance methods, recommended two quart empty metal paint cans for collecting the feces. The cans come with tight-fitting lids and can be purchased in appropriate sizes from any of the hardware stores catering to the paint industry. The empty can is inserted into the toilet bowl and the patient is asked to make sure that the stools fall into the metal can and, if possible, the urine is excluded from the collection. The cans have tight-fitting lids and therefore they can be used for shaking and homogenization of the feces. We have also used these cans and they were quite satisfactory. However, we now prefer to use empty plastic cartons which are used for packing ice cream, etc., by the dairies. These plastic cartons also come in different sizes and have tight-fitting lids. In order to stabilize and hold these cartons in place, we use aluminum sheets in the middle of which a hole is cut to accommodate the carton shown in figure 13. The aluminum sheet is placed over the porcelain toilet bowl but under the plastic or wood seat. Thus, the carton fits within the toilet bowl without projecting unduly upwards and can be used without any discomfort. After use, the cartons or the cans are closed with lids and stored at −20 °C. Alternatively, the cartons can be left at 4 °C for a day or two within which time they are homogenized and aliquots are taken for storage at −20 °C, thus avoiding storage of the bulky cans.

As a general rule, feces are collected in 3-day pools, but it should be possible to obtain equally satisfactory results with 1- or 2-day pools, if markers such as chromic oxide and β-sitosterol are used.

Homogenization

The tin cans generally vary in their weights enough that it is essential to weigh each can before the feces are collected. On the other hand, there is much less variation in the weights of plastic cartons and it is not necessary to weigh each carton before collecting the feces. The cartons or the cans are weighed (again) after fecal collection and the weight of the feces is determined. Unless the feces are unusually liquid, an equal amount of distilled water (by weight) is added to obtain a homogenate that is liquid enough for pipetting out known values of the homogenate. If the metal paint cans are used,

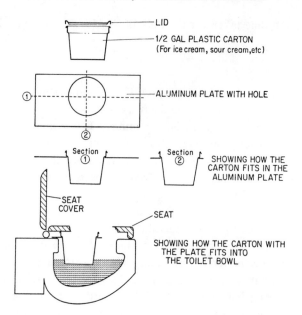

Fig. 13. Description of a simple device for quantitative collection of feces for cholesterol balance studies.

it is recommended that three 2-inch metal washers should be put in each can after it is weighed. This helps in homogenization which is carried out by vigorous agitation for 3–5 min in a paint mixer. The mixture in plastic cartons can be homogenized with a homogenizer (e. g. polytron), thus avoiding the need of metal washers or the paint mixers.

Aliquots of the homogenates are transferred to 125-ml glass bottles (with plastic screw caps) either directly or with the help of wide mouth transfer pipettes. Aliquots must be taken immediately and before the suspended solids have the time to settle out. Contents such as chromic oxide, having a greater density than water, can settle very rapidly; therefore, maximum speed is necessary for collecting the representative samples. If a homogenizer is used (for a number of samples), it should be thoroughly cleaned with water, chloroform methanol, and again with water between homogenizations.

Homogenization of Diet

In order to determine the exact intake of cholesterol and plant sterols, random samples of complete 1-day diets are taken and homogenized in an electric blender. The solid and the liquid components of the diet are pooled together in a large electric blender and homogenized. We have found it to be more convenient to transfer this partially homogenized food to plastic cartons and to subject this to further homogenization with a polytron homogenizer. Aliquots are taken and stored as in the case of feces.

Collection of Blood

Since it is necessary to relate the SA of plasma cholesterol to the SA of metabolites of endogenous cholesterol in feces, the blood samples are taken 2–3 times a week for determining the SA of cholesterol.

Quantitative Isolation of Neutral and Acidic Steroids from Feces

The methods described below for the isolation, purification, and quantitation of acidic and neutral steroids in feces are those developed in Dr. *Ahren*'s laboratory at Rockefeller University [178, 296]. The methods described below differ only in minor details from the methods reported in the original publications.

Monitoring

The extraction, isolation and the determinations of dietary and fecal constituents by procedures listed below may be attended with small but significant losses despite careful techniques. It is therefore advisable to employ markers and standards to correct losses whenever possible. When processing the dietary samples, a simple addition of radioactive cholesterol and/or β-sitosterol is generally sufficient to monitor and correct for the methodological losses. Fecal steroids, however, may already be radioactive, in which case one can add the isotope which is not already present in the feces; i.e. if the fecal steroids already contain ^{14}C, one can add ^{3}H to monitor the losses, and vice versa, into the feces or their extracts. However, care has to be taken especially for samples which exhibit considerable quenching. By adding ^{14}C to monitor the methodological losses of fecal metabolites labeled with ^{3}H, the ability to accurately determine the ^{3}H counts may be significantly compromised. On the other hand, endogenous radioactivity itself may also be used to monitor the methodological losses. Recovery of radioactivity present in total extracts can be used to correct for losses during the TLC of fecal neutral or acidic steroids. The use of β-sitosterol and hyocholic acid or nordeoxycholic acid can also be helpful when they are added (in known amounts)

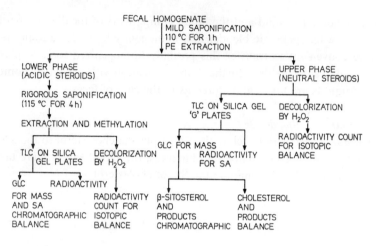

Fig. 14. Flow diagram.

at the beginning of the procedures; their recoveries can be used to correct for the methodological losses [131, 179, 454].

If proper care and precautions are taken during the extraction of the sample of feces, the losses (in the extraction procedure) are generally negligible. However, it may be desirable to establish this by the use of total oxidatio of the solid sample to collect $^{14}CO_2$ or ^3H_2O and compare their activity with the activity in the lipid extracts.

Isolation and Quantitation of Fecal Neutral Steroids

Approximately 1–2 g of fecal homogenate is transferred into a pre-weighed 125-ml reagent bottle and the exact weight of the homogenate is determined. A few boiling chips and 20 ml of N NaOH in 95% alcohol are added, and the sample is refluxed for 1 h at 110–120 °C (fig. 14). After the sample has cooled to room temperature, 10 ml of distilled water and 50 ml of PE (BP 60–70 °C) are added and the mixture is shaken vigorously for 1 min. The phases are allowed to separate (for more rapid separation, the mixture is centrifuged at 1,000 g for 5 min) and the upper PE phase is removed with the help of suction into a 1,000-ml round-bottom flask. The PE extraction is repeated twice and the residue saved for the extraction of bile acids. The pooled extracts are evaporated to dryness in a rotary evaporator and the residue is immediately redissolved in 10 ml of PE.

Estimation of Neutral Steroids by Isotopic Balance

A known aliquot of the PE extract (2–5 ml) is transferred to a stoppered centrifuge and the pigments are bleached by adding 1–2 ml of 30% H_2O_2. Sometimes, it may be necessary to treat the sample with small amounts of H_2O_2 for 24 h to decrease the pigments to acceptable levels. Neutral steroids are reextracted with PE, transferred to a counting vial, evaporated to dryness under a stream of nitrogen, and the radioactivity determined after adding scintillation fluid. The vials should be kept in the dark for at least ½ h and samples counted long enough to get a total of 4,000–10,000 counts. Correcions for background radioactivity and quenching are applied before estimating disintegration rates.

The endogenous fecal neutral steroids are determined by dividing the total radioactivity in the neutral steroid fraction by the SA of plasma cholesterol at the time when the former were secreted in the bile. These data are then corrected for variations in fecal flow and other methodological or biological losses, if any.

To determine total neutral steroids present in feces, whether derived from endogenous cholesterol or from unabsorbed dietary cholesterol, divide the total radioactivity in the fecal extract (of neutral steroids) by the SA of the fecal cholesterol (or of fecal coprostanol).

Quantitation of Fecal Neutral Steroids by Chromatographic Methods

Determine the total radioactivity present in the extract as described in the previous section and use this information to correct for methodological losses during the subsequent procedure. Take an aliquot (3–5 ml) of the PE extract of the fecal neutral steroids and evaporate it to dryness under nitrogen. Reconstitute the lipids in 0.2–0.5 ml of PE and transfer the sample quantitatively to thin-layer plates coated with silica gel G and impregnated with 0.01% rhodamine 6G. Rhodamine 6G can also be sprayed after the development of chromatograms. Another dye that can be sprayed after the chromatograms are developed is $2',7'$-dichlorofluorescein in methanol. Occasionally, when fecal samples contain a lot of fat, the transfer of fecal-neutral steroids to thin-layer plates is made difficult by formation of jelly-like soaps. This difficulty can be overcome by equilibrating the PE phase with 50% ethanol in a centrifuge tube and discarding the lower phase after centrifugation. Losses of neutral steroids in the discarded material can be corrected by the use of radioactive standards.

The samples are applied as a thin streak near the bottom of thin-layer plates, and reference standards of cholesterol, coprostanol, and coprostanone

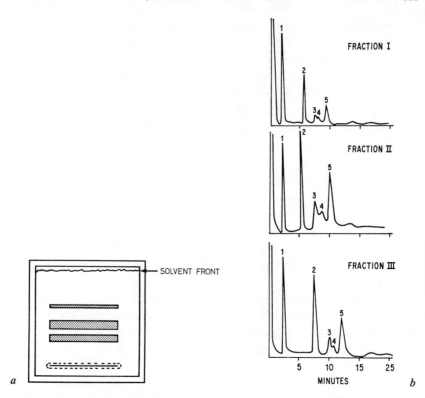

Fig. 15. a TLC separation of fecal neutral steroids. The three bands contain copro-stanone (I), coprostanol (II), and cholesterol (III) as well as the corresponding compounds of plant sterols as shown in (b). *b* GLC separation of fecal neutral steroids. The three fractions (I, II and III) are the same as shown in (a). The first peak in each fraction represents 5α-cholestane, the internal standard. The other peaks represent: fraction I: (2) coprostanone, (3), campestanone (4), stigmastanone, and (5) β-sitostanone; fraction II: (2) coprostanol (3) campestanol, (4) stigmastanol, and (5) β-sitostanol; fraction III: (2) cholesterol, (3) campesterol, (4) stigmasterol, and (5) β-sitosterol.

are spotted on either side of this streak. The plate is developed in ethyl ether : heptane (55:45 v/v) to its full length and taken out of the tank to dry. The bands are delineated in the darkness under UV light with the help of spraying reagents (if necessary). The three bands shown in figure 15a correspond to (1) 3-keto derivatives of cholesterol and plant sterols; (2) saturated 5 β derivatives of cholesterol and plant sterols, and (3) cholesterol and plant sterols (fig. 16). The bands are marked as closely as possible with a needle. Usually, TLC of neutral steroid fraction produces three distinct bands;

FECAL STEROIDS

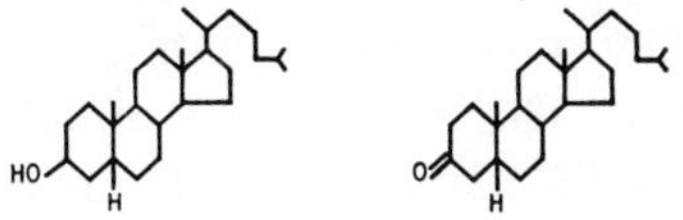

COPROSTANOL   COPROSTANONE

(5β–Cholestan–3β–ol)   (5β–Cholestan–3–one)

Fig. 16. Major microbial degradative products of cholesterol during its transit through the large intestine.

occasionally, however, band 3 may not be visible. (The pattern may also differ if the subject is on antibiotics. Only one band, No. III, is seen in diet samples.) The three bands are scraped individually and without contamination, transferred into sintered glass funnels and eluted with 4 × 5 ml portions of redistilled ethyl ether. The combined ethyl ether eluates are evaporated under nitrogen and the steroids are then dissolved in a known volume of redistilled ethyl acetate (2–5 ml). To one aliquot, a known amount of 5α-cholestane is added (as an internal standard) and then subjected to GLC. Another aliquot is taken for counting and the total recovery in the three bands is used to correct for methodological losses.

GLC of Neutral Steroids

Preparation of silylating reaction mixture. The silylating reagent for the preparation of trimethylsilyl ether (TMS) derivatives of neutral steroids is prepared by mixing N,N-dimethylformamide, hexamethyldisilazane, and tri-methylchlorosilane in proportions of 40:40:1. The mixture is stable for weeks if protected from water vapor.

The aliquot containing 5α-cholestane is transferred into a small, tapered tube and the solvent evaporated to dryness under a stream of nitrogen, sily-lating mixture (0.2 ml/mg of sterol) is added, the tube stoppered and kept at room temperature for 30 min (band 3, i.e. the band containing 3-ketosteroids does not need to be silylated; however, if it is collected with other bands then silylation is necessary for satisfactory separation). The reaction mixture can be immediately subjected to GLC or if the GLC is to be performed later, then it is evaporated and the TMS ethers and 5α-cholestane redissolved in 0.1– 0.2 ml dry ethyl acetate before injection. In practice, it is better to evaporate the silylating reagent and the residue dissolved in ethyl acetate prior to in-jection. This reduces tailing of the solvent front.

Gas-liquid partition chromatography is performed on an instrument equipped with a hydrogen flame ionization detector. Glass columns (4–6 ft) packed with 1% DC560 or 3.8% SE or 3.8% W-98 on acid washed silanized gas chrom P (100–120 mesh) can be used. The temperatures of column, detector and flash heater are maintained at 230, 270, and 300 °C and a carrier gas (nitrogen or helium) flow of 50–60 ml per minute is used. For separation, a known amount (2–3 μl) of ethyl acetate solution is injected into the GLC flash heater. Figure 15b shows typical chromatograms obtained on GLC of fecal neutral steroids.

The mass of the individual components of neutral steroids is calculated from the individual areas of the GLC peaks of the three bands, each relative to the known amount of 5α-cholestane in each sample. Summation of the individual mass will give the total fecal neutral steroid in the injected sample. Total fecal neutral steroids in the homogenate taken for analysis can then be calculated using appropriate factors. The amounts are then corrected for methodological losses and then the daily excretion of fecal neutral steroids are calculated and corrected for fecal flow using chromic oxide recovery data. All the corrections can also be made using data on β-sitosterol recovery.

If endogenous cholesterol is labeled, the SA of fecal cholesterol, coprostanol, and coprostanone can be calculated by dividing the radioactivity in each band by the mass of the steroid in each band.

Isolation and Quantitation of Dietary Steroids
Dietary cholesterol and plant sterols are measured by GLC essentially as described above. For complete recovery of dietary plant sterols, acidic hydrolysis is required since some of the plant sterols apparently are present in ether linkages and cannot be split by alkaline hydrolysis. If this is not taken into consideration, the fecal output of plant sterols may exceed the dietary intake because sterols are deconjugated by bacteria during intestinal passage [295].

Isolation and Quantitation of Acidic Steroids
The lower phase left after removal of fecal neutral steroids is evaporated to near dryness on a water bath or a hot plate and 15 ml of 2 N NaOH added and the contents saponified at 15 psi for 3 h in a pressure cooker. Complete hydrolysis of the conjugated fecal bile acids also could be carried out by refluxing the sample at 115–120 °C for 4 h after adding 15 ml of 2 N NaOH in ethanol. After hydrolysis, the samples are cooled and then acidified to

pH 1–2 with concentrated hydrochloric acid. The sample is then quantitatively transferred to a 125-ml separatory funnel, rinsing out the bottles with 10 ml distilled water and 10 ml of chloroform:methanol (2:1) twice. 30 ml more of chloroform:methanol is added to the separatory funnel, and the mixture shaken for 1 min and the phases allowed to separate. The lower phase is transferred to a 1,000-ml round-bottom flask, and the extraction procedure is repeated twice with 50 ml of chloroform. The pooled extracts are evaporated to dryness and the residue dissolved in a known volume of (10 ml) ethyl acetate.

A known aliquot (5 ml) is then methylated using excess diazomethane in ether. The procedure is repeated to ensure complete methylation. After evaporation of the diazomethane and the ether, the sample is redissolved in 5 ml of ethyl acetate.

Estimation of Fecal Bile Acids
Isotopic Balance
A known volume of (2.5 ml) methylated extract is transferred to a glass-stoppered tube and the sample is decolorized by adding 30% H_2O_2. The bile acids are reextracted with ethyl acetate and the extract is transferred to a counting vial. The solvent is evaporated, counting fluid (PPO-POPOP-toluene) added and the radioactivity (dpm) determined in a liquid scintillation spectrometer.

Total bile acids are estimated by dividing the total radioactivity (dpm) in the acidic steroid fraction by the SA of plasma cholesterol (dpm/mg) 56 h before the midpoint of fecal collections. The data are then corrected for methodological losses and variations in fecal flow.

Chromatographic Balance
A known aliquot of the extract is quantitatively transferred on a thin layer (0,5 mm) of silica gel 'H' plate. Methyl cholate is used as a reference standard. The plate is first developed to the top with benzene, taken out and allowed to dry. The position of the fatty acid methyl esters area (use of fatty acid methyl esters as reference standard will facilitate their identification) is located after exposure to iodine. A line is drawn immediately below the band and the plate is developed for a second time in isooctane:isopropanol:acetic acid (120:40:1 v/v/v) but only up to the line below the fatty acids. After taking the plate out, it is exposed to iodine vapor once again to mark the position of the bile acids. The area containing the bile acids (between the fatty acid band and the methyl cholate band) is scraped and the silica gel

transferred into glass-sintered funnels for elutions with 5×10 ml portions of methanol. The pooled methanol extracts are evaporated and the bile acid methyl esters are redissolved in 5 ml ethyl acetate. A known amount of 5α-cholestane is added to serve as internal standard (not necessary if nordeoxycholic or hyocholic acid is used as a standard at the beginning). An aliquot is counted for determining methodological losses, for estimation of SA and another aliquot is subjected to GLC after trimethylsilylation.

Preparation of TMS of Bile Acids. The bile acid methyl esters are exposed to silylating reagents in order to convert all free hydroxyl groups to TMS ethers. An aliquot of the ethylacetate solution containing bile acid methyl esters and 5α-cholestane standard is transferred into a glass vial of appropriate size. The solvent is evaporated under air with gentle warming. The silylating reagent mixture is added (100 μl/mg or less of mixed bile acid methyl esters), the vial tightly closed and the reaction mixture is left at room temperature for 1 h or longer. The silylating mixture is then evaporated and the sample redissolved in ethyl acetate prior to injection.

Silylating Reagent. Silylating reagent mixture is prepared by mixing pyridine (stored over molecular sieve), hexamethyldisilazene, and trimethylchlorosilane, in proportions of $9:3:1$. The mixture is effective for at least 6 months if protected against contamination by water vapor.

The bile acid TMS, dissolved in ethyl acetate, are injected into GLC column ($1-3$ μl). GLC conditions are identical to those used for fecal neutral steroids. If the quantities of total as well as individual bile acid components are required, then the separation must be done on columns packed with 3% Hi Eff 8B. Alternatively, quantitation of total and individual bile acids could be done on columns packed with 1% QF1 after preparing the trifluoroacetates of bile acid methyl esters. Figure 17 shows typical chromatogram obtained on GLC of fecal acidic steroids.

The area of individual peaks or the total area of all peaks is used to determine the individual or total weight of bile acids relative to 5α-cholestane (or other internal recovery standard). This weight is then corrected for methodological losses on the basis of the recovery of radioactive or other internal standards (bile acids) added at the start of isolation. The data are then corrected for the variations in fecal flow.

We suggest addition of 5α-cholestane to the sample before GLC even if internal standards such as nordeoxycholic and hyocholic acids are used as internal standards. Its addition facilitates identification of the bile acid peaks

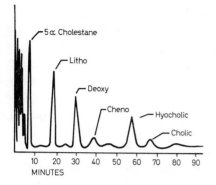

Fig. 17. GLC separation of fecal bile acids as their methyl esters trifluoroacetates on QF-₁column. 5α-cholestane and hyocholic acid are used as internal standards. Other peaks are lithocholic (litho), deoxycholic (deoxy), chenodeoxycholic (cheno), and cholic acids.

since its retention time is shorter than the retention time of the bile acids. GLC determination of fecal bile acids can also be carried out without previous TLC purification provided that the addition of 5α-cholestane (which has to be added) is large enough.

Fecal bile acids have also been estimated by other methods such as fluorometric and enzymatic methods.

Fecal Markers

In metabolic balance studies, stools collected during a given period do not necessarily reflect the biological events that take place in the intestines during the collection period. The flow of the contents from duodenum to the colon and their exit in feces is not always regular. To correct for possible irregularities of the fecal flow, nonabsorbable inert markers are incorporated into the ingested food and their fecal recovery permits the corrections for variations in fecal flow as well as for incomplete collections [238].

A plant sterol such as β-sitosterol makes an ideal marker for cholesterol balance. Chemically, it is very similar in structure to that of cholesterol and its intestinal metabolism (except for its absorption) is almost the same [179, 248]. It has been suggested that identical fractions of β-sitosterol and cholesterol are degraded to non-steroidal compounds by intestinal flora. Since the absorption of β-sitosterol is less than 5% it can be used to correct for the degradative losses of cholesterol in the intestines [179].

Polyethylene glycol has been used frequently as a fecal marker [395, 497]. It is not necessary to administer it for more than a day or two before the studies are begun. Its determination in the feces, however, is tedious and some losses may occur when the fecal sample is stored even at $-20\,^{\circ}C$.

Cromic oxide (Cr_2O_3) is the most widely used marker for the corrections of variations in fecal flow [238, 446]. It is nontoxic, readily measurable, and completely unabsorbable. However, it takes a period of 7–10 days for the chromic oxide to achieve a balance between intake and output. Occasionally, there are subjects who may be less ideal excretors of chromic oxide and *Davignon et al.* [105] suggest that such subjects should be excluded from metabolic studies. On the other hand, *Kottke and Subbiah* (237] showed that the data could be corrected even if the excretion of chromic oxide is as low as 30%. Our experience is also similar to these investigators.

Determination of Chromic Oxide (Cr_2O_3)

A number of methods such as flame spectrophotometry, atomic absorption spectrometry, and color reaction with diphenyl semicarbazide are available for the estimation of Cr_2O_3 in feces [13, 94, 498]. Use of radioactive chromic oxide ($^{51}Cr_2O_3$) has also been made [105]. However, the most commonly used method is the colorimetric method of *Bolin et al.* [51] and this is described below.

Preparation of Oxidizing Agent. Dissolve 10 g of sodium molybdate in 150 ml distilled water. Slowly add 150 ml concentrated sulphuric acid, cool and add 200 ml of perchloric acid (70–72%) and mix thoroughly.

Method. Shake the fecal sample *thoroughly* and transfer about 1–2 g of fecal homogenate containing 1–5 mg of Cr_2O_3 into a thick wall digestion flask calibrated at 25 ml. Note the weight of the homogenate accurately. Add 5 ml of the oxidizing reagent in such a manner that it will wash adhering particles down the side of the flask. Heat the flask to 215 °C. This could be done using heating block or electric digestion rack or microburners. Digest the sample until a clear solution is obtained. Cool slightly; wash down any black particles adhering to the sides or neck of the flask with 2 ml perchloric acid (70–72%). Reheat for another 5 min. Cool and slowly add distilled water to make up the volume to 25 ml. Read the resultant yellow (dichromate) solution at 440 nm in a spectrophotometer. If any insoluble inorganic salts remain in suspension they could be removed by filtration or centrifugation at 3,000 rpm for 10 min.

A standard calibration curve is prepared by oxidizing known amounts of chromic oxide. The contents are diluted to a known volume with distilled water. Different aliquots of this solution are further diluted to 25 ml volume (to give different concentration of chromic oxide) and the color read at 400 nm.

The method is rapid, simple and accurate. The procedures should be carried out in a fumehood and proper precautions should be taken to avoid explosions.

Technologic advances and ingenuity led to the availability of many good methods for the study of cholesterol metabolism and further progress in this field can be anticipated.

References

1   Abaurre, R.; Gordon, S. G.; Mann, J. G., and Kern, F., jr.: Fasting bile salt pool size and composition after ileal resection. Gastroenterology *57:* 679–688 (1969).

2   Abell, L.L.; Levy, B.B.; Brodie, B.B., and Kendall, F.E.: A simplified method for the estimation of total cholesterol in serum and demonstration of its specificity. J. biol. Chem. *195:* 357–366 (1952).

3   Ackerman, M.E.; Redd, W.L.; Tormaneu, C.D.; Hardgrave, J.E., and Scallen, T.J.: The quantitative assay of 3-hydroxy-3-methyl glutaryl coenzyme A reductase: comparison of a thin-layer chromatographic assay with a rapid chloroform extraction assay. J. Lipid Res. *18:* 408–413 (1977).

4   Adams, E. and Baxter, M.: Lipid fractions of human adrenals. Archs Path. *48:* 13–26 (1949).

5   Ahrens, E.H., jr.: The use of liquid formula diets in metabolic studies: 15 years' experience. Adv. metab. Dis. *4:* 297–332 (1970).

6   Ahrens, E.H., jr.: The management of hyperlipidemia: whether, rather than how. Ann. intern. Med. *85:* 87–93 (1976).

7   Ahrens, E.H., jr.; Dole, V.P., and Blankenhorn, D.H.: The use of orally fed liquid formulas in metabolic studies. Am. J. clin. Nutr. *2:* 336–342 (1954).

8   Akanuma, Y.; Yokoyama, S., and Iwasaki, Y.: Plasma lecithin: cholesterol acyl transferase (LCAT) activity of familial type II hyperlipoproteinemias. Proc. 4-th Int. Symp. on Atherosclerosis, Tokyo 1976, p. 234.

9   Albers, R.W. and Lowry, O.H.: Flurometric determination of 0.1 to 10 micrograms of cholesterol. Analyt. Chem. *27:* 1829–1831 (1955).

10   Ali, S.S. and Javitt, N.B.: Quantitative estimation of bile salts in serum. Can. J. Biochem. *48:* 1054–1057 (1970).

11   Allain, C.C.; Poon, L.S.; Chan, C.S.G.; Richmond, W., and Fu, P.C.: Enzymatic determination of total serum cholesterol. Clin. Chem. *20:* 470–475 (1974).

12   Allan, R.N.; Thistle, J.L., and Hofmann, A.F.: Lithocholate metabolism during chemotherapy for gallstone dissolution. II. Absorption and sulfation. Gut *17:* 413–419 (1976).

13   Allen, T.L.: Microdetermination of chromium with 1,5-diphenylcarbo-hydrazide. Analyt. Chem. *30:* 447–450 (1958).

14   Anderson, J.M. and Dietschy, J.M.: Regulation of sterol synthesis in 16 tissues of rat. I. Effect of diurnal light cycling, fasting, stress, manipulation of enterohepatic circulation and administration of chylomicrons and triton. J. biol. Chem. *252:* 3646–3651 (1977).

15   Anthony, W.L. and Beher, W.T.: Color detection of bile acids using thin-layer chromatography. J. Chromat. *13:* 567–570 (1964).

16 Ashworth, L.A.E. and Green, C.: The uptake of lipids by human α-lipoproteins. Biochim. biophys. Acta *70:* 68–74 (1963).

17 Austad, W.I.; Lack, L., and Tyor, M.P.: Importance of bile acids and of an intact distal small intestine for fat absorption. Gastroenterology *52:* 638–646 (1967).

18 Avigan, J.: A method for incorporating cholesterol and other lipids into serum lipoproteins *in vitro*. J. biol. Chem. *234:* 787–790 (1959).

19 Avigan, J.; Goodman, D.S., and Steinberg, D.: Thin-layer chromatography of sterols and steroids. J. Lipid Res. *4:* 100–101 (1963).

20 Avigan, J.; Bhathena, S.J., and Schreiner, M.E.: Control of sterol synthesis and hydroxymethylglutaryl CoA reductace in skin fibroblasts grown from patients with homozygous type II hyperlipoproteinemia. J. Lipid Res. *16:* 151–154 (1975).

21 Bachorik, P.S. and Rogers, A.I.: The direct fluorometric assay of conjugated bile acids. J. Lab. clin. Med. *74:* 705–714 (1969).

22 Back, P.; Hamprecht, B., and Lynen, F.: Regulation of cholesterol biosynthesis in rat liver: diurnal changes of activity and influence of bile acids. Archs Biochem. Biophys. *133:* 11–21 (1969).

23 Balasubramaniam, S.; Mitropoulos, K.A., and Myant, N.B.: Evidence for the compartmentation of cholesterol in rat-liver microsomes. Eur. J. Biochem. *34:* 77–83 (1973).

24 Barter, P.J.: Origin of esterified cholesterol transported in the very low density lipoproteins of human plasma. J. Lipid Res. *15:* 11–19 (1974).

25 Barter, P.J.: Production of plasma esterified cholesterol in lean, normotriglyceridemic humans. J. Lipid Res. *15:* 234–242 (1974).

26 Beg, Z.H.; Allmann, D.W., and Gibson, D.M.: Modulation of 3-hydroxy-3-methylglutaryl coenzyme A reductase activity with CAMP and with protein fractions of rat liver cytosol. Biochem. biophys. Res. Commun. *54:* 1362–1369 (1973).

27 Beher, W.T.; Lin, G.J., and Strandnieks, S.: A rapid flexible method for determining bile lipids. Henry Ford Hosp. med. J. *23:* 87–104 (1975).

28 Benjamin, A.; Pourfar, M., and Schneck, L.: Automated chromatography for stepwise elution of complex lipids. J. Lipid Res. *10:* 616–618 (1969).

29 Bennett, R.D. and Heftmann, E.: Thin-layer chromatography of sterols. J. Chromat. *9:* 359–362 (1962).

30 Bergström, S. and Danielsson, H.: Formation and metabolism of bile acids; in Code, Handbook of physiology, Vol. V, pp. 2391–2407 (Am. Physiological Society, Washington 1968).

31 Bergström, S.: The formation of bile acids from cholesterol in the rat. Fysiografiska, Sallskapets *22:* 1–5 (1952).

32 Bergström, S. and Samuelson, B.: in Lundberg Autooxidation and antioxidants, vol. I, pp. 233–248 (Interscience, New York 1961).

33 Bergström S. and Danielsson, H.: On the regulation of bile acid formation in the rat liver. Acta physiol. scand. *43:* 1–7 (1958).

34 Berthelot, M.: Sur plusieurs alcools nouveaux. Annls Chim. physiol. *56:* 51–98 (1859).

35 Bhattacharyya, A.K. and Connor, W.E.: β-Sitosterolemia and xanthomatosis: a newly described lipid storage disease in two sisters. J. clin. Invest. *53:* 1033–1043 (1974).

36 Bhattacharyya, A.; Connor, W.E., and Spector, A.A.: Excretion of sterols from skin of normal and hypercholesterolemic humans. J. clin. Invest. *51:* 2060–2070 (1972).

37 Bierman, E.L.; Stein, O., and Stein, Y.: Lipoprotein uptake and metabolism by rat aortic smooth muscle cells in tissue culture. Circulation Res. *35:* 136–150 (1974).

38 Bills, C.E.: Physiology of sterols including vitamin D. Physiol. Rev. *15:* 1–97 (1935).

39 Björkhem, I. and Danielsson, H.: Assay of liver microsomal cholesterol 7α-hydroxylase using deuterated carrier and gas chromatography mass spectrometry. Analyt. Biochem. *59:* 508–516 (1974).

40 Björkhem, I. and Danielsson, H.: 7α-Hydroxylation of exogenous and endogenous cholesterol in rat liver microsomes. Eur. J. Biochem. *53:* 63–70 (1975).

41 Blandon, P.: Chemistry; in Cook, Cholesterol: chemistry, biochemistry and pathology, pp. 15–115 (Academic Press, New York 1958).

42 Bloch, K.: The biological conversion of cholesterol to pregnanediol. J. biol. Chem. *157:* 661–666 (1945).

43 Bloch, K.: The biological synthesis of cholesterol. Science *150:* 19–28 (1965).

44 Bloch, K.; Berg, B.N., and Rittenberg, D.: The biological conversion of cholesterol to cholic acid. J. biol. Chem. *149:* 511–517 (1943).

45 Block, W.D.; Jarret, K.J., and Levine, J.B.: Use of a single colour reagent to improve the automated determination of serum total cholesterol; in Skeggs, Automation in analytical chemistry, pp. 345–347 (Mediad, New York 1965).

46 Blomhoff, J.P.: Serum cholesterol determination by gas-liquid chromatography. Clin. chim. Acta *43:* 257–265 (1973).

47 Blomhoff, J.P.: *In vitro* determination of lecithin: cholesterol acyltransferase activity in plasma. Scand. J. clin. Lab. Invest. *33:* suppl. 137, pp. 35–43 (1974).

48 Blomstrand, R. and Ahrens, E.H., jr.: The absorption of fats studied in a patient with chyluria III cholesterol. J. biol. Chem. *233:* 327–330 (1958).

49 Bloor, W.R.: The determination of small amounts of lipids in blood plasma. J. biol. Chem. *77:* 53–73 (1928).

50 Bloor, W.R. and Knudson, A.: Cholesterol and cholesterol esters in human blood. J. biol. Chem. *29:* 7–13 (1917).

51 Bolin, D.W.; King, R.P., and Klosterman, E.W.: A simplified method for the determination of chromic oxide (Cr_2O_3) when used as an index substance. Science *116:* 634–635 (1952).

52 Bondjers, G. and Bjorkerud, S.: Fluorimetric determination of cholesterol and cholesteryl esters in tissue on nanogram level. Analyt. Biochem. *42:* 363–371 (1971).

53 Borgström, B.: Investigation on lipid separation methods: separation of phospholipids from neutral fat and fatty acids. Acta physiol. scand. *25:* 101–110 (1952).

54 Borgström, B.: Investigation on lipid separation methods: separation of cholesterol esters, glycerides and free fatty acids. Acta physiol. scand. *25:* 110–118 (1952).

55 Borgström, B.: Studies on intestinal cholesterol absorption in the human. J. clin. Invest. *39:* 809–815 (1960).

56 Borgström, B.: Quantitative aspects of the intestinal absorption and metabolism of cholesterol and β-sitosterol in the rat. J. Lipid Res. *9:* 473–481 (1968).

57 Borgström, B.: Quantification of cholesterol absorption in man by fecal analysis after the feeding of a single isotope labelled meal. J. Lipid Res. *10:* 331–337 (1969).

58   Borgström, B.: Bile salts–their physiological functions in the gastrointestinal tract. Acta med. scand. *196:* 1–10 (1974).

59   Borgström, B.; Lindhe, B.A., and Wlodawer, P.: Absorption and distribution of cholesterol-4-C14 in the rat. Proc. Soc. exp. Biol. Med. *99:* 365–368 (1958).

60   Borgström, B.; Radner, S., and Werner, B.: Lymphatic transport of cholesterol in the human being. Effect of dietary cholesterol. Scand. J. clin. Lab. Invest. *26:* 227–235 (1970).

61   Borkowski, A.; Delcroix, C., and Levin, S.: Metabolism of adrenal cholesterol in man. I. *In vivo* studies. J. clin. Invest. *51:* 1664–1678 (1972).

62   Boyd, E.M.: The extraction of lipids from the red blood cells. J. biol. Chem. *115:* 37–45 (1966).

63   Boyd, E.M.: Species variation in normal plasma lipids estimated by oxidative micromethods. J. biol. Chem. *143:* 131–132 (1942).

64   Boyd, G.S. and Oliver, M.F.: The physiology of the circulating cholesterol and lipoproteins; in Cook, Cholesterol: chemistry, biochemistry and pathology, p. 181 (Academic Press, New York 1958).

65   Boyd, G.S.; Eastwood, M.A., and Maclean, N.: Bile acids in the rat: studies in experimental occlusion of the bile duct. J. Lipid Res. *7:* 83–94 (1966).

66   Bricker, L.A.; Kozlovskis, P.L., and Goodman, M.G.: Negative feedback in sterol biosynthesis and lipoprotein relase by the perfused rat liver. Proc. Soc. exp. Biol. Med. *143:* 375–378 (1973).

67   Brooks, C.J.W. and Keates, R.A.B.: Gel filtration in lipophilic solvents using hydroxyalkoxypropyl derivatives of Sephadex. J. Chromat. *44:* 509–521 (1969).

68   Brooks, C.J.W. and Smith, A.G.: Cholesterol oxidase: further studies of substrate specificity in relation to the analytical characterization of steroids. J. Chromat. *112:* 499–511 (1975).

69   Brown, M.S. and Goldstein, J.L.: Receptor-mediated control of cholesterol metabolism. Science *191:* 150–154 (1976).

70   Brown, M.S.; Dana, S.E., and Goldstein, J.L.: Regulation of 3-hydroxy-3-methylglutaryl coenzyme A reductase activity in human fibroblasts by lipoproteins. Proc. natn. Acad. Sci. USA *70:* 2162–2166 (1973).

71   Bruusgaard, A.: Quantitative determination of the major 3-hydroxy bile acids in biological material after thin-layer chromatographic separation. Clin. chim. Acta *28:* 495–504 (1970).

72   Bucher, N.L.R.; Overath, P., and Lynen, F.: β-Hydroxymethylglutaryl coenzyme A reductase cleavage and condensing enzymes in relation to cholesterol formation in rat liver. Biochim. biophys. Acta *40:* 491–501 (1960).

73   Burchard, H.: Beitrage zur Kenntniss der Cholesterine; diss., Rockstock (1889).

74   Burstein, M. and Scholnick, H.R.: Precipitation of chylomicrons and very low density lipoproteins from human serum with sodium lauryl sulfate. Life Sci. *11:* 177–184 (1972).

75   Burstein, M. and Scholnick, H.R.: Lipoprotein-polyanion-metal interactions. Adv. Lipid Res. *11:* 67–108 (1973).

76   Burstein, M.; Scholnick, H.R., and Morfin, R.: Rapid method for the isolation of lipoproteins from human serum by precipitation with polyanions. J. Lipid Res. *11:* 583–595 (1970).

77 Byers, S.O. and Friedman, M.: Observations concerning the production and excretion of cholesterol in mammals. XIII. Role of chylomicra in transport of cholesterol and lipid. Am. J. Physiol. *179:* 79–84 (1954).

78 Carroll, K.K.: Separation of lipid classes by chromatography on Florisil. J. Lipid Res. *2:* 135–141 (1961).

79 Carroll, K.K.: Acid treated Florisil as an adsorbent for column chromatography. J. Am. Oil Chem. Soc. *40:* 413–419 (1963).

80 Cham, B.E. and Knowles, B.R.: A solvent system for delipidation of plasma or serum without protein precipitation. J. Lipid Res. *17:* 176–181 (1976).

81 Cham, B.E.; Hurwood, J.J.; Knowles, B.R., and Powell, L.W.: Rapid, sensitive method for the separation of free cholesterol from ester cholesterol. Clin. chim. Acta *49:* 109–113 (1973).

82 Chevallier, F.: Dynamics of cholesterol in rats, studied by the isotopic equilibrium method. Adv. Lipid Res. *5:* 209–239 (1967).

83 Chevreul, M.E.: Recherches chimiques sur plusieurs corps gras, et particulièrement sur leurs combinations avec les alcalis. Cinquième mémoire. Des corps qu'on a appelés adipocise, c'est-á-dire, de la substance cristallisée des calculs biliaires humains, du spermacéti et de la substance grasse de cadavres. Annls Chim. *95:* 5–50 (1815).

84 Chevreul, M.E.: Sixième mémoire. Examen des graisses d'homme, de mouton, de bœuf, de jagar et de oie. Annls Chim. Phys. *2:* 339–372 (1816).

85 Chobanian, A.V.; Burrows, B.A., and Hollander, W.: Body cholesterol metabolism in man. II. Measurement of the body cholesterol miscible pool and turnover rate. J. clin. Invest. *41:* 1738–1744 (1962).

86 Clifton-Bligh, P.; Miller, N.E., and Nestel, P.J.: Increased plasma cholesterol esterifying activity during colestipol resin therapy in man. Metabolism *23:* 437–444 (1974).

87 Clinkenbeard, K.D.; Sugiyama, T.; Moss, J.; Reed, W.D., and Lane, M.D.: Molecular and catalyitc properties of cytosolic acetoacetyl coenzyme A thiolase from avian liver. J. biol. Chem. *248:* 2275–2284 (1973).

88 Clinkenbeard, K.D.; Reed, W.D.; Mooney, R.A., and Lane, M.D.: Intracellular localization of the 3-hydroxy-3-methyl coenzyme A cycle enzymes in liver. J. biol. Chem. *250:* 3108–3116 (1975).

89 Connor, W.E.; Witiak, D.T.; Stone, D.B., and Armstrong, M.L.: Cholesterol balance and fecal neutral steroid and bile acid excretion in normal men fed dietary fats of different fatty acid composition. J. clin. Invest. *48:* 1363–1375 (1969).

90 Cook, R.P.: Distribution of sterols in organisms and in tissues; in Cook, Cholesterol: chemistry, biochemistry and pathology, pp. 145–180 (Academic Press, New York 1958).

91 Cowen, A.E.; Korman, M.G.; Hofmann, A.F., and Cass, O.W.: Metabolism of lithocholate in healthy man. I. Biotransformation and biliary excretion of intravenously administered lithocholate, litholcholyl glycine and their sulfates. Gastroenterology *69:* 59–66 (1975).

92 Cronholm, T. and Sjövall, J.: Bile acids in portal blood of rats fed different diets and cholestyramine. Bile acids and steroids 189. Eur. J. Biochem. *2:* 374–383 (1967).

93 Crouse, J.R.: Validation of a new out-patient method for measuring cholesterol absorption in man. Circulation 55: suppl. III, p. 186 (1977).

94 Daly, J.R. and Anstall, H.B.: The determination of chromium sesquioxide in faeces by flame spectrometry. Clin. chim. Acta 9: 576–580 (1964).

95 Daly, M.M.: Biosynthesis of squalene and sterols by rat aorta. J. Lipid Res. 12: 367–375 (1971).

96 Dam, H.: Historical introduction; in Cook, Cholesterol: chemistry, biochemistry and pathology, pp. 1–14 (Academic Press, New York 1958).

97 Danielsson, H. and Einarsson, K.: The enzymic formation of 7α-hydroxycholesterol from cholesterol in rat liver homogenates. Acta chem. scand. 18: 831–832 (1964).

98 Danielsson, H. and Einarsson, K.: Formation and metabolism of bile acids; in The biological basis of medicine, vol. 5, pp. 279–315 (Academic Press, New York 1969).

99 Danielsson, H. and Gustafsson, B.: On serum cholesterol levels and neutral fecal sterols in germ-free rats. Bile acids and steroids 59. Archs Biochem. 83: 482–485 (1959).

100 Danielsson, H. and Sjövall, J.: Bile acid metabolism. Annu. Rev. Biochem. 44: 233–253 (1975).

101 Danielsson, H.; Insull, W., jr.; Jordan, P., and Strand, O.: Metabolism of 4-C14-cholesterol in the isolated perfused rat liver. Am. J. Physiol. 202: 699–702 (1962).

102 Danielsson, H.; Eneroth, P.; Hellstrom, K.; Lindstedt, S., and Sjovall, J.: On the turnover and excretory products of cholic and chenodeoxycholic acid in man. J. biol. Chem. 238: 2299–2304 (1963).

103 Darmady, E.M. and Davenport, S.G.T.: Hematological technique, pp. 181–182 (Grune & Stratton, New York 1954).

104 David, J.S.K.; Soloff, L.A., and Lacko, A.G.: Factors affecting esterification of lipoprotein cholesterol by lecithin: cholesterol acyl transferase. Life Sci. 18: 701–706 (1976).

105 Davignon, J.; Simmonds, W.J., and Ahrens, E.H., jr.: Usefulness of chromic oxide as an internal standard for balance studies in formula fed patients and for assessment of colonic function. J. clin. Invest. 47: 127–137 (1968).

106 Davis, R.A.; Showalter, P.J., and Kern, F., jr.: Measurement of bile acid synthesis by 14CO2: the metabolism of propionyl CoA. Steroids 26: 408–421 (1975).

107 Fourcroy De: De la substance feuilletée et cristalline contenue dans les calculs biliaires, et de la nature des concrétions cystiques cristalisées. Ann. Chim. 3: 242–252 (1789).

108 Delsal, J.L.: Microdosages colorimétriques du choléstérol libre, du choléstérol estérifié et du phosphore lipidique dans le liquide céphalorachidien. C.r. Séanc Soc. Biol. 141: 268–269 (1947).

109 Dempsey, M.E.: Cholesterol biosynthesis in vitro. Hypolipidemic agents; in Kritchevsky. Handbook of experimental pharmacology, vol. 41, pp. 1–28 (Springer, Berlin 1975).

110 Denbesten, L.; Connor, W.E.; Kent, T.H., and Lin, D.: Effect of cellulose in the diet on the recovery of dietary plant sterols from the feces. J. Lipid Res. 11: 341–345 (1970).

111 Souza, N.J. De and Nes, W.R.: Improved separation of sterols by reversed-phase thin-layer chromatography. J. Lipid Res. 10: 240–243 (1969).

112 Dietschy, J.M.: The mechanism of the intestinal absorption of bile acids. J. Lipid Res. *9:* 297–309 (1968).

113 Dietschy, J.M. and Siperstein, M.D.: Effect of cholesterol feeding and fasting on sterol synthesis in seventeen tissues of the rat. J. Lipid Res. *8:* 97–104 (1967).

114 Dietschy, J.M. and Wilson, J.D.: Cholesterol synthesis in the squirrel monkey: relative rates of synthesis in various tissues and mechanisms of control. J. clin. Invest. *47:* 166–174 (1968).

115 Dietschy, J.M. and Wilson, J.D.: Regulation of cholesterol metabolism. Parts 1 to 3. New Engl. J. Med. *282:* 1128–1138, 1179–1183, 1241–1249 (1970).

116 Dietschy, J.M. and Gamel, W.G.: Cholesterol synthesis in the intestine of man. Regional differences and control mechanisms. J. clin. Invest. *50:* 872–880 (1971).

117 Dietschy, J.M.; Weeks, L.E., and Delente, J.J.: Enzymatic mesurement of free and esterified cholesterol esters in plasma and other biological preparations using the oxygen electrode in a modified glucose analyzer. Clin. chim. Acta *73:* 407–414 (1976).

118 Downing, D.T.: Photodensitometry in the thin-layer chromatographic analysis of neutral lipids. J. Chromat. *38:* 91–99 (1968).

119 Doyle, J.T.; Dawber, T.R.; Kannel, W.B.; Kinch, S.H., and Kahn, H.A.: The relationship of cigarette smoking to coronary heart disease. J. Am. med. Ass. *190:* 886–890 (1964).

120 Driscoll, J.L.; Aubuchon, D.; Descoteux, M., and Martin, H.F.: Semiautomated specific routine serum cholesterol determination by gas liquid chromatography. Analyt. Chem. *43:* 1196–1200 (1971).

121 Duane, W.C.; Adler, R.D.; Bennion, L.J., and Ginsberg, R.L.: Determination of bile acid pool size in man: a simplified method with advantages of increased precision, shortened analysis time and decreased isotope exposure. J. Lipid Res. *16:* 155–158 (1975).

122 Durr, I.F. and Rudeny, H.: The reduction of β-hydroxy-β-methyl-glutarly coenzyme A to mevalonic acid. J. biol. Chem. *235:* 2572–2578 (1960).

123 Eastwood, M.A.; Hamilton, D., and Mowbray, L.: A method for the estimation of bile acid conjugates and bile acids in biological fluids. J. Chromat. *65:* 407–411 (1972).

124 Eckles, N.E.; Taylor, C.B.; Campbell, D.J., and Gould, R.G.: The origin of plasma cholesterol and the rates of equilibration of liver, plasma and erythrocyte cholesterol. J. Lab. clin. Med. *46:* 359–371 (1955).

125 Edelman, I.S. and Liebman, J.: Anatomy of body water and electrolytes. Am. J. Med. *27:* 256–277 (1959).

126 Edwards, P.A.; Muroya, H.H., and Gould, R.G.: *In vivo* demonstration of the circadian rhythm of cholesterol biosynthesis in the liver and intestines of the rat. J. Lipid Res. *13:* 396–401 (1972).

127 Einarsson, K.; Hellstrom, K., and Kallner, M.: Randomly tritium-labelled chenodeoxycholic acid as tracer in the determination of bile acid turnover. Clin. chim. Acta *56:* 235–239 (1974).

128 Ellingboe, J.; Nyström, E., and Sjovall, J.: Liquid gel chromatography on lipophilic hydrophobic Sephadex derivatives. J. Lipid Res. *11:* 266–273 (1970).

129 Eneroth, P.: Thin-layer chromatography of bile acids. J. Lipid Res. *4:* 11–16 (1963).

130 Eneroth, P.; Gordon, B.; Ryhage, R., and Sjovall, J.: Identification of mono- and

dihydroxy bile acids in human feces by gas liquid chromatography and mass spectrometry. J. Lipid Res. 7: 511–523 (1966).

131 Evrard, E. and Janssen, G.: Gas liquid chromatographic determination of human fecal bile acids. J. Lipid Res. 9: 226–236 (1968).

132 Ewing, A.M.; Freeman, N.K., and Lindgren, F.T.: The analysis of human serum lipoprotein distributions. Adv. Lipid Res. 3: 25–61 (1965).

133 Faergeman, O. and Havel, R.J.: Metabolism of cholesteryl esters of rat very low density lipoproteins. J. clin. Invest. 55: 1210–1218 (1975).

134 Fausa, O. and Skalhegg, B.A.: Quantitative determination of bile acids and their conjugates using thin layer chromatography and a purified 3β-hydroxysteroid dehydrogenase. Scand. J. Gastroent. 9: 249–254 (1974).

135 Fawcett, J.K. and Wynn, V.: Effects of posture on plasma volume and some blood constituents. J. clin. Path. 13: 304–310 (1960).

136 Fieser, L.F.: A companion of cholesterol. J. Am. chem. Soc. 73: 5007 (1951).

137 Fieser, L.F.: Cholesterol and companions. III. Cholestanol, lathosterol and ketone 104. J. Am. chem. Soc. 75: 4395–4403 (1953).

138 Fieser, L.F.: Cholesterol and companions. VII. Steroid dibromides. J. Am. chem. Soc. 75: 5421–5422 (1953).

139 Fieser, L.F.: Some aspects of the chemistry and biochemistry of cholesterol. Science 119: 710–716 (1954).

140 Fieser, L.F. and Fieser, M.: Natural products related to phenanthrene; 3rd ed. (Reinhold, New York 1949).

141 Fillerup, D.L. and Mead, J.F.: Chromatographic separation of plasma lipids. Proc. Soc. exp. Biol. 83: 574–577 (1953).

142 Fimognari, G.M. and Rodwell, V.W.: Mevalonate biosynthesis in rat liver. Lipids 5: 104–108 (1970).

143 Flegg, H.M.: An investigation of the determination of serum cholesterol by an enzymatic method. Ann. clin. Biochem. 10: 79–84 (1973).

144 Fogleman, A.M.; Edmond, J.; Polito, A., and Popjak, G.: Control of lipid metabolism in human leukocytes. J. biol. Chem. 248: 6928–6929 (1973).

145 Folch, J.; Ascoli, I.; Lees, M.; Meath, J.A., and LeBaron, F.N.: Preparation of lipid extracts from brain tissue. J. biol. Chem. 191: 833–841 (1951).

146 Folch, J.; Lees, M., and Sloane-Stanley, G.H.: A simple method for the isolation and purification of total lipids from animal tissues. J. biol. Chem. 226: 497–509 (1957).

147 Forman, D.T.; Phillips, C.; Eiseman, W., and Taylor, C.B.: Fluorimetric measurement of fecal bile acids. Clin. Chem. 14: 348–359 (1968).

148 Fredrickson, D.S.; Levy, R.I., and Lees, R.S.: Fat transport in lipoproteins: an integrated approach to mechanisms and disorders. New Engl. J. Med. 276: 34–44, 94–103, 148–156, 215–225, 273–281 (1967).

149 Gadez, T.R.; Allan, R.N.; Mach, E., and Hofmann, A.F.: Impaired lithocholate sulfation in the rhesus monkey: a possible mechanism for chenodeoxycholate toxicity. Gastroenterology 70: 1125–1129 (1976).

150 Gänshirt, V.H.; Koss, F.W., and Moranz, K.: Untersuchung zur quantitativen Auswertung der Dunnschichtchromatographie. Arzneimittel-Forsch. 10: 943–947 (1960).

151 Gidez, L.I.; Roheim, P.S., and Eder, H.A.: Turnover of cholesteryl esters of plasma lipoproteins in the rat. J. Lipid Res. 8: 7–15 (1967).

152 Glomset, J.A.: The mechanism of the plasma cholesterol esterification reaction and plasma fatty acid transferase. Biochim. biophys. Acta *65:* 128–135 (1962).

153 Glomset, J.A.: The plasma lecithin: cholesterol acyltransferase reaction. J. Lipid Res. *9:* 144–167 (1968).

154 Glomset, J.A.: Physiological role of lecithin–cholesterol acyl-transferase. Am. J. clin. Nutr. *23:* 1129–1136 (1970).

155 Glomset, J.A. and Wright, J.L.: Some properties of a cholesterol esterifying enzyme in human plasma. Biochim. biophys. Acta *89:* 266–276 (1964).

156 Glomset, J.A.; Janssen, F.T.; Kennedy, R., and Dobbins, J.: Role of plasma lecithin: cholesterol acyltransferase in the metabolism of high density lipoproteins. J. Lipid Res. *7:* 638–648 (1966).

157 Gloster, J. and Fletcher, R.F.: Quantitaitve analysis of serum lipids with thin-layer chromatography. Clin. chim. Acta *13:* 235–240 (1966).

158 Glover, J.; Green, C., and Stainer, D.W.: Sterol metabolism. 5. The uptake of sterols by organelles of intestinal mucosa and the site of their esterification during absorption. Biochem. J. *72:* 82–87 (1959).

159 Glover, M.; Glover, J., and Morton, R.A.: Provitamin D_3 in tissues and the conversion of cholesterol to 7-dehydrocholesterol *in vivo*. Biochem. J. *51:* 1–9 (1952).

160 Goldfarb, S. and Pitot, H.C.: Improved assay of 3-hydroxy-3-methyl glutaryl coenzyme A reductase. J. Lipid Res. *12:* 512–515 (1971).

161 Goldrick, R.B. and Hirsch, J.: A technique for quantitative recovery of lipids from chromatoplates. J. Lipid Res. *4:* 482–483 (1963).

162 Goldstein, J.L. and Brown, M.S.: Lipoprotein receptors cholesterol metabolism and atherosclerosis. Archs Path. *99:* 181–184 (1975).

163 Goodman, D.S.: The metabolism of chylomicron cholesterol ester in the rat. J. clin. Invest. *41:* 1886–1896 (1962).

164 Goodman, D.S.: Cholesterol ester metabolism. Physiol. Rev. *43:* 747–839 (1965).

165 Goodman, D.S. and Shiratori, T.: *In vivo* turnover of different cholesterol esters in rat liver and plasma. J. Lipid Res. *5:* 578–586 (1964).

166 Goodman, D.S. and Noble, R.P.: Turnover of plasma cholesterol in man. J. clin. Invest. *47:* 231–241 (1968).

167 Goodman, D.S.; Noble, R.P., and Dell, R.B.: Three pool model of the long-term turnover of plasma cholesterol in man. J. Lipid Res. *14:* 178–188 (1973).

168 Goodwin, C.D. and Margolis, S.: Improved methods for the study of hepatic HMG CoA reductase: one step isolation of mevalonolactone and rapid preparation of endoplasmic reticulum. J. Lipid Res. *17:* 294–303 (1976).

169 Goswami, S.K. and Frey, C.F.: A novel method for the separation and identification of bile acids and phospholipids of bile on thin-layer chromatograms. J. Chromat. *89:* 87–91 (1974).

170 Gould, R.G.: Symposium on sitosterol. IV. Absorbability of beta sitosterol. Trans. N.Y. Acad. Sci. *18:* 129–134 (1955).

171 Gould, R.G. and Popjak, G.: Biosynthesis of cholesterol *in vivo* and *in vitro* from DL-β-hydroxy-β-methyl-δ-[2-C^{14}] valerolactone. Biochem. J. *66:* 51 (1957).

172 Gould, R.G.; Taylor, C.B.; Hagerman, J.S.; Warner, I., and Campbell, D.J.: Cholesterol metabolism. I. Effect of dietary cholesterol on the synthesis of cholesterol in dog tissue *in vitro*. J. biol. Chem. *201:* 519–528 (1953).

173 Gould, R.G.; Le Roy, G.V.; Okita, G.T.; Kabara, J.J.; Keegan, P., and Bergenstal, D.M.: Use of C14 labelled acetate to study cholesterol metabolism in man. J. Lab. clin. Med. *46:* 374–384 (1955).
174 Gregg, J.A.: New solvent systems for thin layer chromatography of bile acids. J. Lipid Res. *7:* 579–581 (1966).
175 Grundy, S.M. and Ahrens, E.H., jr.: An evaluation of the relative merits of two methods for measuring the balance of sterols in man: isotopic balance versus chromatographic analysis. J. clin. Invest. *45:* 1503–1515 (1966).
176 Grundy, S.M. and Ahrens, E.H., jr.: Measurements of cholesterol turnover, synthesis and absorption in man, carried out by isotope kinetic and sterol balance methods. J. Lipid Res. *10:* 91–107 (1969).
177 Grundy, S.M. and Metzger, A.L.: A physiological method for estimation of hepatic secretion of biliary lipids in man. Gastroenterology *62:* 1200–1217 (1972).
178 Grundy, S.M.; Ahrens, E.H., jr., and Miettinen, T.A.: Quantitative isolation and gas-liquid chromatographic analysis of total fecal bile acids. J. Lipid Res. *6:* 397–410 (1965).
179 Grundy, S.M.; Ahrens, E.H., jr., and Salen, G.: Dietary β-sitosterol as an internal standard to correct for cholesterol losses in sterol balance studies. J. Lipid Res. *9:* 374–387 (1968).
180 Grundy, S.M.; Ahrens, E.H., jr., and Davignon, J.: The interaction of cholesterol absorption and cholesterol synthesis in man. J. Lipid Res. *10:* 304–315 (1969).
181 Grundy, S.M.; Ahrens, E.H., jr., and Salen, G.: Interruption of the enterohepatic circulation of bile acids in man. Comparative effects of cholestyramine and ileal exclusion on cholesterol metabolism. J. Lab. clin. Med. *78:* 94–121 (1971).
182 Gurpide, E.; Mann, J., and Lieberman, S.: Analysis of open systems of multiple pools by administration of tracers at a constant rate or as a single dose as illustrated by problems involving steroid hormones. J. clin. Endocr. Metab. *23:* 1155–1176 (1963).
183 Gurpide, E.; Mann, J., and Sandberg, E.: Determination of kinetic parameters in a two-pool system by administration of one or more tracers. Biochemistry, N.Y. *3:* 125–1255 (1964).
184 Haahthi, E.; Nikkari, T., and Juva, K.: Fractionation of serum and skin sterol esters and skin waxes with chromatography on silica gel impregnated with silver nitrate. Acta chem. scand. *17:* 538–540 (1963).
185 Hadley, G.G. and Weiss, S.P.: Further notes on use of salts of ethylene diamine tetra-acetic acid (EDTA) as anticoagulants. Am. J. clin. Path. *25:* 1090–1093 (1955).
186 Haeckel, R. and Perlick, M.: A new enzymatic determination of cholesterol. The use of aldehyde dehydrogenase to measure H_2O_2 producing reactions. II. J. clin. Chem. clin. Biochem. *14:* 411–414 (1976).
187 Hagerman, J.S. and Gould, R.G.: The *in vitro* interchange of cholesterol between plasma and red cells. Proc. Soc. exp. Biol. Med. *78:* 329–332 (1951).
188 Ham, A.B.: A new reagent for the determination of true cholesterol. Am. J. med. Technol. *37:* 319–324 (1971).
189 Hamilton, J.G.: The effect of oral neomycin on the conversion of cholic acid to deoxycholic in man. Archs Biochem. Biophys. *101:* 7–13 (1963).
190 Hamilton, W.F.; Moore, J.W.; Kinsman, J.M., and Spurling, R.G.: Studies on the

circulation. IV. Further analysis of the injection method, and of changes in hemodynamics under physiological and pathological conditions. Am. J. Physiol. *99:* 534–551 (1932).

191 Hamprecht, B.; Nüssler, C., and Lynen, F.: Rhythmic changes of hydroxymethylglutaryl Coenzyme A reductase activity in livers of fed and fasted rats. FEBS Lett. *4:* 117–121 (1969).

192 Hanahan, D.J.; Watts, R.M., and Pappajohn, D.: Some chemical characteristics of the lipids of human and bovine erythrocytes and plasma. J. Lipid Res. *1:* 421–432 (1960).

193 Harris, P.A. and Harris, K.L.: Quantitative GLC analysis of plasma cholesterol. J. pharm. Sci. *63:* 781–784 (1974).

194 Hatch, F.T. and Lees, R.S.: Practical methods for plasma lipoprotein analysis. Adv. Lipid Res. *6:* 1–68 (1968).

195 Heaton, K.W.; Austad, W.I.; Lack, L., and Tyor, M.P.: Enterohepatic circulation of ^{14}C labeled bile salts in disorders of distal small bowel. Gastroenterology *55:* 5–16 (1968).

196 Hechter, O.; Solomon, M.M.; Zaffaroni, A., and Pincus, G.: Transformation of cholesterol and acetate to adrenal cortical hormones. Archs Biochem. *46:* 201–213 (1953).

197 Hele, P.: The acetate activating enzyme of beef heart. J. biol. Chem. *206:* 671–676 (1954).

198 Heller, V.G. and Paul, H.: Changes in cell volume produced by varying concentrations of different anticoagulants. J. Lab. clin. Med. *19:* 777–782 (1934).

199 Hellman, L.; Rosenfeld, R.S.; Insull, W.R., and Ahrens, E.H., jr.: Intestinal excretion of cholesterol: a mechanism for regulation of plasma levels. J. clin. Invest. *36:* 898a (1957).

200 Hepner, G.W.; Hofmann, A.F., and Thomas, P.J.: Metabolism of steroid and amino acid moieties of conjugated bile acids in man. I. Cholylaglycine. J. clin. Invest. *51:* 1889–1897 (1972).

201 Hernandez, H.H.; Peterson, D.W.; Chaikoff, I.L., and Dauben, D.W.: Absorption of cholesterol-4-^{14}C in rats fed mixed soybean sterols and ß-sitosterol. Proc. Soc. exp. Biol. Med. *83:* 498–499 (1953).

202 Hesse, O.: Über Phytosterin und Cholesterin. Ann. *192:* 175–179 (1878).

203 Hirsch, J. and Ahrens, E.H., jr.: The separation of complex lipide mixtures by the use of silicic acid chromatography. J. biol. Chem. *233:* 311–320 (1958).

204 Hislop, I.G.; Hofmann, A.F., and Schoenfield, L.J.: Determinants of the rate and site of bile acid absorption in man. J. clin. Invest. *46:* 1070–1071 (1967).

205 Hoff, H.F.; Jackson, R.L.; Mao, J.T., and Gotto, A.M.: Localization of low density lipoproteins in arterial lesions from normolipemics employing a purified fluorescent labeled antibody. Biochim. Biophys. Acta *351:* 407–415 (1974).

206 Hoffman, N.E.; LaRusso, N.F., and Hofmann, A.F.: Sampling intestinal content with a sequestering capsule: a noninvasive technique for determining bile acid kinetics in man. Mayo Clin. Proc. *51:* 171–175 (1976).

207 Hofmann, A.F.: Thin-layer adsorption chromatography of free and conjugated bile acids on silicic acid. J. Lipid Res. *3:* 127–128 (1962).

208 Hofmann, A.F.: The function of bile salts in fat absorption. The solvent properties of dilute micellar solutions of conjugated bile salts. Biochem. J. 89: 57–68 (1963).

209 Hofmann, A.F.: Thin-layer chromatography of bile acids and their derivatives; in Morris and James, New biochemical separations, pp. 261–282 (Van Nostrand, London 1964).

210 Hofmann, A.F.: A physiochemical approach to the intraluminal phase of fat absorption. Gastroenterology 50: 56–64 (1966).

211 Hofmann, A.F. and Small, D.M.: Detergent properties of bile salts: correlation with physiological function. Annu. Rev. Med. 18: 333–376 (1967).

212 Hofmann, A.F. and Hoffman, N.E.: Measurement of bile acid kinetics by isotope dilution in man. Gastroenterology 67: 314–323 (1974).

213 Hofmann, A.F.; Schoenfield, L.J.; Kotke, B.A., and Poley, J.R.: Methods for the description of bile acid kinetics in man; in Methods in medical research, vol. 12, pp. 149–180 (Year Book, Chicago 1970).

214 Holman, R.T.: Autoxidation of fats and related substances; in Holman, Lundberg and Malkins, Progress in the chemistry of fats and other lipids, vol. 2, pp. 51–58 (Pergamon Press, Oxford 1954).

215 Horlick, L.; Kudchodkar, B.J., and Sodhi, H.S.: Mode of action of chlorophenoxyisobutyric acid on cholesterol metabolism in man. Circulation 43: 299–309 (1971).

216 Hoshita, A. and Ohigashi, T.: The metabolism of bile acids. VII. On the metabolism of bile acids in the pigeon intestine. Hiroshima J. med. Sci. 9: 111–117 (1960).

217 Huang, T.C.; Chen, C.P.; Wefler, V., and Raftery, A.: A stable reagent for the Libermann-Burchard reaction. Analyt. Chem. 33: 1405–1407 (1961).

218 Huang, T.L. and Nichols, B.L.: New solvent systems for the separation of free and conjugated bile acids. J. Chromat. 101: 235–239 (1974).

219 Huber, J.; Latzin, S., and Hamprecht, B.: A simple and rapid radiochemical assay for 3-hydroxy-3-methylglutaryl coenzyme A reductase. Hoppe-Seyler's Z. physiol. Chem. 354: 1645–1647 (1973).

220 Hürthle, K.: Über die Fettsäure-cholesterin-ester des Blutserums. Hoppe-Seyler's Z. physiol. Chem. 21: 331–359 (1896).

221 Ikekawa, N.; Matusi, M., and Sato, K.: Simultaneous determination of cholesterol and cholesterol esters in serum by gas chromatography. Jap. J. exp. Med. 41: 163–170 (1971).

222 Iritani, N. and Nogi, J.: Cholesterol absorption and lymphatic transport in rat. Atherosclerosis 15: 231–239 (1972).

223 Ishikawa, T.T.; MacGee, J.; Morrison, J.A., and Glueck, C.J.: Quantitative analysis of cholesterol in 5 to 20 microliters of plasma. J. Lipid Res. 15: 286–291 (1974).

224 Iwata, T. and Yamasaki, K.: Enzymic determination and thin layer chromatography of bile acids in blood. J. Biochem., Tokyo 56: 424–431 (1974).

225 Johnson, D.B.; Tyor, M.P., and Lack, L.: The use of [7α-³H] and [7α7β-³II] cholesterol in the enzymic assay of cholesterol 7α-hydroxylase. J. Lipid Res. 17: 353–359 (1976).

226 Johnston, J.M.: Mechanisms of fat absorption; in Code, Handbook of physiology, vol. 3, pp. 1353–1376 (Williams & Wilkins, Baltimore 1968).

Jones, M.E.; Black, S.; Flynn, R.M., and Lipmann, F.: Acetyl coenzyme A synthesis
227 through pyrophosphoryl split of ATP. Biochim. biophys. Acta 12: 141–149 (1953).

228 Kaihara, S. and Wagner, H.N.: Measurement of intestinal fat absorption with carbon-14 labeled tracers. J. Lab. clin. Med. 71: 400–411 (1968).

229 Kamel, A.M.; Felmeister, A., and Weiner, N.D.: Surface pressure surface area characteristics of a series of autoxidation products of cholesterol. J. Lipid Res. 12: 155–159 (1971).

230 Kammereck, R.; Lee, W.H.; Paliokas, A., and Schroepfer, G.J., jr.: Thin layer chromatography of sterols on neutral alumina impregnated with silver nitrate. J. Lipid Res. 8: 282–284 (1967).

231 Kandutsch, A.A. and Saucier, S.E.: Prevention of cyclic and triton-induced increases in hydroxy-methyl-glutaryl coenzyme A reductase and sterol synthesis by puromycin. J. biol. Chem. 244: 2299–2305 (1969).

232 Kannel, W.B.; Dawber, T.R.; Friedman, C.D.; Glennon, W.E., and McNamara, P.M.: An evaluation of several serum lipids as predictors of coronary heart disease. The Framingham study. Ann. intern. Med. 61: 888–899 (1964).

233 Keys, A.: Coronary heart diesease – the global picture. Atherosclerosis 22: 149–192 (1975).

234 Kim, E. and Goldberg, M.: Serum cholesterol assay using a stable Lieberman-Burchard reagent. Clin. Chem. 15: 1171–1179 (1969).

235 Koerselman, H.B.; Lewis, B., and Pilkington, T.R.E.: The effect of venous occlusion on the level of serum cholesterol. J. Atheroscler. Res. 1: 85–88 (1961).

236 Kottke, B.A.: Differences in bile acid excretion. Primary hypercholesterolemia compared to combined hypercholesterolemia and hypertriglyceridemia. Circulation 40: 13–20 (1969).

237 Kottke, B.A. and Subbiah, M.T.R.: Sterol balance studies in patients on solid diets. Comparison of two nonabsorbable markers. J. Lab. clin. Med. 86: 530–538 (1972).

238 Kreula, M.S.: Absorption of carotene from carrots in man and the use of the quantitative chromic oxide indicator method in the absorption experiments. Biochem J. 41: 269–273 (1947).

239 Kritchevsky, D.: Biochemistry of steroids; in Schettler, Lipid and lipidoses, pp. 66–92 (Springer, Berlin 1967).

240 Kritchevsky, D. and Kirk, M.R.: Detection of steroids in paper chromatography. Archs Biochem. Biophys. 35: 346–351 (1952).

241 Kritchevsky, D.; Martak, D.S., and Rothblat, G.H.: Detection of bile acids in thin layer chromatography. Analyt. Biochem. 5: 388–392 (1963).

242 Kritchevsky, D.; Tepper, S.A., and Story, J.A.: Non-nutritive fiber and lipid metabolism. J. Food Sci. 40: 8–11 (1975).

243 Kritchevsky, D.; Davidson, L.M.; Kim, H.K., and Malhotra, S.: Quantitation of serum lipids by a simple TLC-charring method. Clin. chim. Acta 46: 63–68 (1973).

244 Kudchodkar, B.J. and Sodhi, H.S.: Turnover of plasma cholesteryl esters and its relationship to other parameters of lipid metabolism in man. Eur. J. clin. Invest. 6: 285–298 (1976).

245 Kudchodkar, B.J. and Sodhi, H.S.: Plasma cholesteryl esters turnover in man: comparison of in vivo and in vitro methods. Clin. chim. Acta 68: 187–194 (1976).

246 Kudchodkar, B.J.; Sodhi, H.S., and Horlick, L.: Comparison of isotopic and gas-liquid chromatographic methods for cholesterol balance studies in man. Clin. Res. 19: 4A (1971).

247 Kudchodkar, B.J.; Sodhi, H.S., and Horlick, L.: Comparison of isotopic and chromatographic methods for estimating fecal bile acids. Clin. chim. Acta 41: 47–54 (1972).

248 Kudchodkar, B.J.; Sodhi, H.S., and Horlick, L.: Lack of degradation of dietary and endogenous sterols in gastrointestinal tract of man. Metabolism 21: 343–349 (1972)

249 Kudchodkar, B.J.; Sodhi, H.S., and Horlick, L.: Absorption of dietary cholesterol in man. Metabolism 22: 155–163 (1973).

250 Kudchodkar, B.J.; Sodhi, H.S.; Horlick, L., and Mason, D.T.: Mechanism of hypocholesterolemic effect of nicotinic acid in man. Clin. Pharmac. Ther. 24: 354–373 (1978).

251 Kuksis, A.: Newer developments in determination of bile acids and steroids by gas chromatography; in Glick, Methods of biochemical analysis, vol. 14, pp. 326–454 (Interscience, New York 1966).

252 Kuksis, A. and Beveridge, J.M.R.: The paper chromatographic fractionation of plant steryl esters. Can. J. Biochem. Physiol. 38: 95–106 (1960).

253 Kuksis, A. and Huang, T.C.: Differential absorption of plant sterols in the dog. Can. J. Biochem. 40: 1493–1504 (1962).

254 Kuksis, A.; Marai, L., and Gornall, D.A.: Direct gas chromatographic examination of total lipid extracts. J. Lipid Res. 8: 352–357 (1967).

255 Kuksis, A.; Myher, J.J.; Marai, L., and Geher, K.: Determination of plasma lipid profiles by automated gas chromatography and computerized data analysis. J. Chromat. Sci. 13: 423–430 (1975).

256 Kumar, A. and Christian, G.D: Enzymatic assay of total cholesterol in serum or plasma by amperometric measurement of rate of oxygen depletion following saponification. Clin. chim. Acta 74: 101–108 (1977).

257 Labarrére, J.A.; Chipault, J.R., and Lundburg, W.O.: Cholesteryl esters of long-chain fatty acids infra-red spectra and separation by paper chromatography. Analyt. Chem. 30: 1466–1470 (1958).

258 LaRusso, N.F.; Hoffman, N.E., and Hofmann, A.F.: Validity of using 2,4-^{3}H-labeled bile acids to study bile acid kinetics in man. J. Lab. clin. Med. 84: 759–765 (1974).

259 Lester, D.: Determination of acetic acid in blood and other tissues by vacuum distillation and gas-liquid chromatography. Analyt. Chem. 36: 1810–1812 (1964).

260 Levin, S. J.; Irvin, J.L., and Johnston, C.G.: Spectrofluorometric determination of total bile acids in bile. Analyt. Chem. 33: 856–860 (1961).

261 Lewis, R. and Gorbach, S.: Modification of bile acids by intestinal bacteria. Archs intern. Med. 130: 545–549 (1972).

262 Liebermann, C.: Über das Oxychinoterpen. Ber. 18: 1803–1809 (1885).

263 Lindgren, F.T.: Preparative ultracentrifugal laboratory procedures and suggestions for lipoprotein analysis; in Perkins Analysis of lipids and lipoproteins, pp. 204–224 (Am. Oil Chemists' Society, 1975).

264 Lindgren, F.T.; Jensen, L.C., and Hatch, F.T.: The isolation and quantitative analysis of serum lipoproteins; in Nelson, Blood lipids and lipoproteins, quantitation, composition and metabolism, pp. 181–274 (Wiley-Inserscience, New York 1972).

265 Lindstedt, S.: The turnover of cholic acid in man. Acta physiol. scand. 40: 1–9 (1957).

266 Lipid Research Clinics Program: Manual of laboratory operations. Department of Health, Education and Welfare handbook, vol. 1, pp. 75–628 (1974).

267 Lippman, A.E.; Foltz, E.W., and Djerassi, C.: Optical rotation dispersion studies. III. The cholestane series. J. Am. chem. Soc. 77: 4364–4367 (1955).

268 Liu, G.C.K.; Ahrens, E.H., jr.; Schreibman, P.H.; Samuel, P.; McNamara, D.J., and Crouse, J.R.: Measurement of cholesterol synthesis in man by isotope kinetics of squalene. Proc. nat. Acad. Sci. USA 72: 4612–4616 (1975).

269 Liu, G.C.K.; Ahrens, E.H., jr.; Schreibman, P.H., and Crouse, J.R.: Measurement of squalene in human tissues and plasma: validation and application. J. Lipid Res. 17: 38–45 (1976).

270 Lossow, W.J.; Brot, N., and Chaikoff, I.L.: Disposition of cholesterol moiety of a chylomicron containing lipoprotein fraction of chyle in the rat. J. Lipid Res. 3: 207–215 (1962).

271 Lynen, F.: Lipid metabolism. Annu. Rev. Biochem. 24: 653–688 (1955).

272 Lynen, F.: Biosynthesis. Terpenes, sterols. Ciba Found. Symp. 1958, pp. 95–118 (1959).

273 MacDonald, I.; Williams, C.N., and Mahony, D.E.: A 3α-7α-hydroxy-steroid dehydrogenase assay for conjugated dihydroxy-bile acid mixtures. Analyt. Biochem. 57: 127–136 (1974).

274 MacDonald, I.A.; Williams, C.N., and Mahony, D.E.: Lyophilized 7α-hydroxy-steroid dehydrogenase: a stable enzyme preparation for routine bile acid analysis. J. Lipid Res. 16: 244–246 (1975).

275 MacDonald, I.A.; Williams, C.N., and Mahony, D.E.: A rapid non-chromatographic analysis of individual bile acids in human bile extraction. J. theor. Biol. 57: 385–389 (1976).

276 MacGee, J.; Ishikawa, T.; Miller, W.; Evans, G.; Steiner, P., and Glueck, C.J.: A micromethod for analysis of total plasma cholesterol using gas-liquid chromatography. J. Lab. clin. Med. 82: 656–662 (1973).

277 Mak, K.M. and Trier, J.S.: Radioautographic and chemical evidence for [5-³H]-mevalonate incorporation into cholesterol by rat villous absorptive cells. Biochim. biophys. Acta 280: 316–328 (1972).

278 Makino, I. and Sjövall, J.: A versatile method for analysis of bile acids in plasma. Anal. Lett. 5: 341–349 (1972).

279 Makino, I.K.; Shinozaki, K., and Nakagawa, S.: Sulfated bile acid in urine of patients with hepatobiliary diseases. Lipids 8: 47–49 (1973).

280 Makino, I; Shinozaki, K., and Nakagawa, S.: Measurement of sulfated and non-sulfated bile acids in human serum and urine. J. Lipid Res. 15: 132–138 (1974).

281 Malinow, M.R.; McLaughlin, P.; Papworth, L., and Kittinger, G.W.: A new method for determining liver microsomal cholesterol 7α-hydroxylase. Steroids 25: 663–672 (1975).

282 Mangold, H.K.: Thin layer chromatography of lipids. J. Am. Oil chem. Soc. 38: 708–727 (1961).

283 Mangold, H.K. and Malins, D.C.: Fractionation of fats, oils and waxes on thin layers of silicic acid. J. Am. Oil Chem. Soc. 37: 383–385 (1960).

284 Marcel, Y.L. and Vezina, C.: A method for the determination of the initial rate of reaction of lecithin: cholesterol acyltransferase in human plasma. Biochim. biophys. Acta 306: 497–504 (1973).

References   151

285 Marsh, J.B. and Weinstein, D.B.: Simple charring method for determination of lipids. J. Lipid Res. 7: 574–576 (1966).
286 Maurizi, C.P.; Alvarez, C.; Fischer, G.C., and Taylor, C.B.: Human tissue cholesterol. Archs Path. 86: 644–646 (1968).
287 Maxwell, M.A.B. and Williams, J.P.: The purification of lipid extracts using Sephadex LH-20. J. Chromat. 31: 62–68 (1967).
288 McNamara, D.J.; Ahrens, E.H., jr.; Samuel, P., and Crouse, J.R.: Measurement of daily cholesterol synthesis rates in man by assay of the fractional conversion of mevalonic acid to cholesterol. Proc. natn. Acad. Sci. USA 74: 3043–3046 (1977).
289 Miettinen, M.; Karvonen, M.J.; Turpeinen, O.; Elosno, R., and Paavilainen, E.: Effect of cholesterol lowering diet on mortality from coronary heart disease and other causes. Lancet ii: 835–838 (1972).
290 Miettinen, T.A.: Effect of dietary cholesterol and cholic acid on cholesterol synthesis in rat and man. Prog. biochem. Pharmacol., vol. 4, pp. 68–70 (Karger, Basel 1968).
291 Miettinen, T.A.: Serum squalene and methyl sterols as indicators of cholesterol synthesis in vivo. Life Sci. 8: 713–721 (1969).
292 Miettinen, T.A.: Detection of changes in human cholesterol metabolism. Ann. clin. Res. 2: 300–320 (1970).
293 Miettinen, T.A.: Serum methyl sterols and their distribution between major lipoprotein fractions in different clinical conditions. Ann. clin. Res. 3: 264–271 (1971).
294 Miettinen, T.A.: Bile acid metabolism; in Kritschevsky, Hypolipidemic agents. Handbook of experimental pharmacology, vol. 41, pp. 109–150 (Springer, Berlin 1975).
295 Miettinen, T.A.: Methods for evaluation of hypolipidemic drugs in man: mechanism of their action; in Paoletti and Glueck, Lipid pharmacology, vol. 2, pp. 83–125 (Academic Press, New York 1976).
296 Miettinen, T.A.; Ahrens, E.H., jr., and Grundy, S.M.: Quantitative isolation and gas liquid chromatographic analysis of total dietary and fecal neutral steroids. J. Lipid Res. 6: 411–424 (1965).
297 Miller, G.J. and Miller, N.E.: Plasma-high-density-lipoprotein concentration and development of ischemic heart disease. Lancet i: 16–19 (1975).
298 Miller, W.L., jr. and Baumann, C.A.: Skin steroids. IV. Distribution of Δ7-cholesterol Proc. Soc. exp. Biol. Med. 85: 561–564 (1954).
299 Mitropoulos, K.A. and Myant, N.B.: The metabolism of cholesterol in the presence of liver mitochondria from normal and thyroxine treated rats. Biochem. J. 94: 594–603 (1965).
300 Mitropoulous, K.A. and Myant, N.B.: The formation of lithocholic acid, chenodeoxycholic acid and α-and-β-muricholic acids from cholesterol incubated with rat liver mitochondria. Biochem. J. 103: 472–479 (1967).
301 Mitropoulos, K.A. and Balasubramaniam, S.: Cholesterol 7α-hydroxylase in rat liver microsomal preparations. Biochem. J. 128: 1–9 (1972).
302 Miyake, Y. and Fukuyama, M.: An oxygraphic method for the determination of cholesterol and measurement of the slow oxygen consuming reactions of hepatic microsomes. J. Biochem., Tokyo 79: 613–620 (1976).
303 Mok, H.Y.I. and Dowling, R.H.: How well can we measure bile acid pool size?;

in Matern, Hochensmidt, Bach and Gerak, Advances in bile acid research, pp. 315–332 (Stuttgart, New York 1975).

304 Morin, R.J.: Rapid enzymatic determination of free and esterified cholesterol content of serum and tissues. Clin. chim. Acta 71: 75–80 (1976).

305 Morris, L.J.: Fractionation of cholesterol esters by thin layer chromatography. J. Lipid Res. 4: 357–359 (1963).

306 Morris, L.J.: Separation of lipids by silver ion chromatography. J. Lipid Res. 7: 717–732 (1966).

307 Morris, M.D.; Chaikoff, I.L.; Felts, J.M.; Abraham, S., and Fausa, N.O.: The origin of serum cholesterol in the rat. Diet versus synthesis. J. biol. Chem. 224: 1039–1045 (1957).

308 Mosbach, E.H.: Hepatic synthesis of bile acids. Biochemical steps and mechanisms of rate control. Archs intern. Med. 130: 478–487 (1972).

309 Mukherjee, K.D. and Mangold, H.K.: Recent developments in the chromatographic analysis and purification of radioactively labelled lipids. J. labelled Compds 9: 779–803 (1973).

310 Munster, D.J.; Lever, M., and Carrell, R.W.: Contributions of other sterols to the estimation of cholesterol. Clin. chim. Acta 68: 167–175 (1976).

311 Muroya, H.; Sodhi, H.S., and Gould, R.G.: Sterol synthesis in intestinal villi and crypt cells of rats and guinea pigs. J. Lipid Res. 18: 301–308 (1977).

312 Murphy, G.M.; Billing, B.H., and Baron, D.N.: A fluorimetric and enzymatic method for the estimation of serum total bile acids. J. clin. Path. 23: 594–598 (1970).

313 Murthy, S.K.; David, J.S.K., and Ganguly, J.A.: Some observations on the mechanism of absorption of cholesterol in rat. Biochim. biophys. Acta 70: 490–492 (1963).

314 Myant, N.B. and Lewis, B.: Estimation of the rate of breakdown of cholesterol in man by measurement of $^{14}CO_2$ excretion after intravenous [26-^{14}C] cholesterol. Clin. Sci. 30: 117–127 (1966).

315 Myant, N.B. and Mitropoulos, K.A.: Cholesterol 7α-hydroxylase. J. Lipid Res. 18: 135–153 (1977).

316 Nagasaki, T. and Akanuma, Y.: A new colorimetric method for the determination of plasma lecithin-cholesterol acyltransferase activity. Clin. chim. Acta 75: 371–375 (1977).

317 Nair, P.P.; Gordon, M.; Gordon, S.; Reback, J., and Mendeloff, A.I.: The cleavage of bile acid conjugates by cell-free extracts from Clostridium perfringens. Life Sci. 4: 1887–1892 (1965).

318 Nair, P.P.; Gordon, M., and Reback, J.: The enzymatic cleavage of the carbon-nitrogen bond in 3α, 7α, 12α-trihydroxy-5β-cholan-24-oylglycine. J. biol. Chem. 242: 7–11 (1967).

319 Nelson, G.J.: Studies on the lipids of sheep red blood cells. I. Lipid composition in low and high potassium red cells. Lipids 2: 64–71 (1967).

320 Nelson, G.J.: Handling extraction and storage of blood samples; in Nelson, Blood lipids and lipoproteins quantitation, composition and metabolism, pp. 3–24 (Wiley-Interscience, New York 1972).

321 Ness, A.T.; Pastewka, J.V., and Peacock, A.C.: Evaluation of a recently reported stable Liebermann-Burchard reagent and its use for the direct determination of serum total cholesterol. Clin. chim. Acta 10: 229–237 (1964).

322 Nestel, P.J.: Turnover of plasma esterified cholesterol: influence of dietary fat and carbohydrate and relation of plasma lipids and body weight. Clin. Sci. *38:* 593–600 (1970).

323 Nestel, P.J. and Couzens, E.A.: Turnover of individual cholesterol esters in human liver and plasma. J. clin. Invest. *45:* 1234–1240 (1966).

324 Nestel, P.J. and Monger, E.A.: Turnover of plasma esterified cholesterol in normo-cholesterolemic and hypercholesterolemic subjects and its relation to body build. J. clin. Invest. *46:* 967–974 (1967).

325 Nestel, P.J. and Hunter, J.D.: Differences in bile acid excretion in subjects with hypercholesterolemia, hypertriglyceridemia and overweight. Aust. N.Z. J. Med. *4:* 491–496 (1974).

326 Nestel, P.J. and Kudchodkar, B.J.: Plasma squalene as an index of cholesterol synthesis. Clin. Sci. mol. Med. *49:* 621–624 (1975).

327 Nestel, P.J.; Havel, R.J., and Bezman, A.: Metabolism of constituent lipids of dog chylomicrons. J. clin. Invest. *42:* 1313–1321 (1963).

328 Nestel, P.J.; Whyte, H.M., and Goodman, D.S.: Distribution and turnover of cholesterol in humans. J. clin. Invest. *48:* 982–991 (1969).

329 Nichols, A.V. and Smith, L.: Effect of very low density lipoproteins on lipid transfer in incubated serum. J. Lipid Res. *6:* 206–210 (1965).

330 Nicolau, G.; Shefer, S.; Salen, G., and Mosbach, E.M.: Determination of hepatic 3-hydroxy-3-methylglutaryl CoA reductase activity in man. J. Lipid Res. *15:* 94–98 (1974).

331 Nicolau, G.; Shefer, S.; Salen, G., and Mosbach, E.H.: Determination of hepatic cholesterol 7α-hydroxylase activity in man. J. Lipid Res. *15:* 146–151 (1974).

332 Nicolau, G.; Shefer, S., and Mosbach, E.H.: Determination of microsomal cholesterol by an isotope derivative method. Analyt. Biochem. *68:* 255–259 (1975).

333 Nikkari, T.; Schreibman, P.H., and Ahrens, E.H., jr.: *In vivo* studies of sterol and squalene secretion by human skin. J. Lipid Res. *15:* 563–573 (1974).

334 Nikkari, T.; Schreibman, P.H., and Ahrens, E.H., jr.: Isotopic kinetics of human skin cholesterol secretion. J. exp. Med. *141:* 620–633 (1975).

335 Nilsson, A. and Zilversmit, D.B.: Fate of intravenously injected particulate and lipoprotein cholesterol in the rat. J. Lipid Res. *13:* 32–38 (1972).

336 Noma, A. and Nakayama, K.: Polarographic method for rapid microdetermination of cholesterol with cholesterol esterase and cholesterol oxidase. Clin. Chem. *22:* 336–340 (1976).

337 Norman, A. and Shorb, M.: *In vitro* formation of deoxycholic and lithocholic acid by human intestinal microorganisms. Proc. Soc. exp. Biol. Med. *110:* 552–555 (1962).

338 Norum, K.R. and Gjone, E.: Familal plasma lecithin: cholesterol acyltransferase deficiency – biochemical study of a new inborn error of metabolism. Scand. J. clin Lab. Invest. *20:* 231–243 (1967).

339 Ockner, R.K. and Isselbacher, K.J.: Recent concepts of intestinal fat absorption. Rev. Physiol. Biochem. Pharmacol. *71:* 107–146 (1974).

340 Oliveira, M.M. and Vaughan, M.: Incorporation of fatty acids into phospholipids of erythrocyte membranes. J. Lipid Res. *5:* 156–162 (1964).

341 O'Moore, R.R.L. and Percy-Robb, I.W.: Analysis of bile acids and their conjugates

in jejunal juice by thin layer chromatography and direct densitometry. Clin. chim. Acta *43:* 39–47 (1973).

342 Page, I.H. and Moinuddin, M.: The effect of venous occlusion on serum cholesterol and total protein concentration – a warning. Circulation *25:* 651–652 (1962).

343 Palmer, R.H.: The formation of bile acid sulfates: a new pathway of bile acid metabolism in humans. Proc. natn. Acad. Sci. USA *58:* 1047–1050 (1967).

344 Palmer. R.H.: Bile acids, liver injury and liver disease. Archs intern. Med. *130:* 606–617 (1972).

345 Palmer, R.H. and Bolt, M.D.: Bile acid sulfates. I. Synthesis of lithocholic acid sulfates and their identification in human bile. J. Lipid Res. *12:* 671–679 (1971).

346 Panveliwalla, D.K.; Pertsemlidis, D., and Ahrens, E.H., jr.: Tritiated bile acids: problems and recommendations. J. Lipid Res. *15:* 530–532 (1974).

347 Panzer, T.: Über das sogenannte Protagon der Niere. Hoppe-Seyler's Z. physiol. Chem. *48:* 519–527 (1906).

348 Parekh, A.C. and Jung, D.H.: Cholesterol determination with ferricacetate-uranium acetate and sulfuric acid-ferrous sulfate reagents. Analyt. Chem. *42:* 1423–1427 (1970).

349 Parekh, A.C. and Creno, R.J.: Submicrogram assay of serum and adrenal cholesterol by a simple, direct non-extraction procedure. Biochem. Med. *13:* 241–250 (1975).

350 Parekh, A.C.; Caranto, M.; Mathur, R.K., and Jung, D.H.: Fractionation of serum cholesterol: a critique. Annls clin. Lab. Sci. *6:* 423–429 (1976).

351 Patsch, W.; Sailer, S., and Braunsteiner, H.: An enzymatic method for the determination of the initial rate of cholesterol esterification in human plasma. J. Lipid Res. *17:* 182–185 (1976).

352 Patterson, G.W.; Khalil, M.A., and Idler, D.R.: Sterols of scallop. I. Application of hydrophobic Sephadex derivatives to the resolution of a complex mixture of marine sterols. J. Chromat. *115:* 153–159 (1975).

353 Pearson, S.; Stern, S., and McGavak, T.H.: A rapid accurate method for determination of total cholesterol in serum. Analyt. Chem. *25:* 813–814 (1953).

354 Pelick, N.; Wilson, T.L.; Miller, M.E., and Angeloni, F.M.: Some practical aspects of thin-layer chromatography of lipids. J. Am. Oil Chem. Soc. *42:* 393–399 (1965).

355 Perl, W. and Samuel, P.: Input-output analysis for total input rate and total traced mass of body cholesterol in man. Circulation Res. *25:* 191–199 (1969).

356 Porath, J.R.; Axen, R., and Ernback, S.: Chemical coupling of proteins to agerose. Nature, Lond. *215:* 1491–1492 (1967).

357 Porte, D., jr. and Havel, R.J.: The use of cholesterol-4-^{14}C labeled lipoproteins as a tracer for plasma cholesterol in dog. J. Lipid Res. *2:* 357–362 (1961).

358 Privett, O.S. and Blank, M.L.: Charring condition for quantitative analysis of mono-, di- and triglycerides by thin layer chromatography. J. Am. Oil Chem. Soc. *39:* 520 (1962).

359 Privett, O.S.; Blank, M.D.; Codding, D.W., and Nickell, E.C.: Lipid analysis by quantitative thin layer chromatography. J. Am. Oil Chem. Soc. *42:* 381–391 (1965).

360 Privett, O.S.; Dougherty, K.A., and Castelli, J.D.: Quantitative analysis of lipid classes. Am. J. clin. Nutr. *24:* 1265–1275 (1971).

361 Quintão, E.; Grundy, S.M., and Ahrens, E.H., jr.: An evaluation of four methods for measuring cholesterol absorption by the intestine in man. J. Lipid Res. *12:* 221–232 (1971).

362 Quintão, E.; Grundy, S.M., and Ahrens, E.H., jr.: Effects of dietary cholesterol on the regulation of total body cholesterol in man. J. Lipid Res. *12:* 233–247 (1971).

363 Rabinowitz, J.L. and Gurin, S.: Biosynthesis of cholesterol and β-hydroxy-β-methyl glutaric acid by extracts of liver. J. biol. Chem. *208:* 307–313 (1954).

364 Radin, N.S.: Forisil chromatography. Meth. Enzym. *14:* 268–272 (1969).

365 Radin, N. and Gramza, A.L: Standard of purity for cholesterol. Clin. Chem. *9:* 121–134 (1963).

366 Ray, B.R.; Davisson, E.O., and Crespi, H.L.: Experiments on the degradation of lipoproteins from serum. J. Phys. Chem. *58:* 841–846 (1954).

367 Redgrave, T.G.: Formation of cholesterol esters rich particulate lipid during metabolism of chylomicrons. J. clin. Invest. *49:* 465–471 (1970).

368 Redgrave, T.G. and Dunne, K.B.: Chylomicron formation and composition in unanaesthetized rabbits. Atherosclerosis *22:* 389–400 (1975).

369 Reed, W.D.; Clinkenbeard, K.D., and Lane, M.D.: Molecular and catalytic properties of mitochondrial (ketogenic) 3-hydroxy-3-methylglutaryl coenzyme A synthase of liver. J biol. Chem. *250:* 3117–3123 (1975).

370 Rehnborg, C.S. and Nichols, A.V.: The fate of cholesteryl esters in human serum incubated *in vitro* at 38°. Biochim. biophys. Acta *84:* 596–603 (1964).

371 Richards, R.G.; Mendenhall, C.L., and MacGee, J.: A simple rapid method for measurement of acetate in tissue and serum. J. Lipid Res. *16:* 395–397 (1975).

372 Richmond, W.: Preparation and properties of a cholesterol oxidase from *Nocardia* sp. and its application to the enzymatic assay of total cholesterol in serum. Clin. Chem. *19:* 1350–1356 (1973).

373 Robertson, G. and Cramp, D.G.: An evaluation of cholesterol determinations in serum and serum lipoprotein fractions by a semiautomated fluorimetric method. J. clin. Path. *23:* 243–245 (1970).

374 Roda, A.; Festi, D.; Sama, C.; Mazzella, G.; Aldini, R.; Roda, E., and Barbara, L.: Enzymatic determination of cholesterol in bile. Clin. chem. Acta *64:* 337–341 (1975).

375 Rodwell, V.W.; Nordstrom, J.L., and Mitschelen, J.J.: Regulation of HMG–COA reductase. Adv. Lipid Res. *14:* 1–74 (1976).

376 Roeschlau, P.; Bernet, E. und Gruber, W.: Enzymatische Bestimmung des Gesamtcholesterins in Serum. Z. klin. Chem. klin. Biochem. *12:* 403–407 (1974).

377 Roeschlau, P.; Bernet, E., and Gruber, W.: in Bergmeyer Methods of enzymatic analysis, vol. 4, pp. 1890–1893 (Academic Press, New York 1974).

378 Rose, H.G.: *In vitro* precipitation of particulate radioisotopic cholesterol from human serum. Biochim. biophys. Acta *144:* 686–689 (1967).

379 Rose, H.G.: Origin of cholesteryl esters in the blood of cholesterol-fed rabbits: relative contributions of serum lecithin cholesterol acyltransferase and hepatic ester synthesis. Biochim. biophys. Acta *260:* 312–326 (1972).

380 Rose, H.G. and Juliano, J.: Regulation of plasma lecithin:cholesterol acyltransferase. II. Activation during alimentary lipemia. J. Lab. clin. Med. *89:* 524–532 (1977).

381 Rosenfeld, R.S.; Fukushima, D.K.; Hellman, L., and Gallagher, T.F.: The transformation of cholesterol to coprostanol. J. biol. Chem. *211:* 301–311 (1954).

382 Roseleur, O.J. and Gent, C.M. van: Alkaline and enzymatic hydrolysis of conjugated bile acids. Clin. chim. Acta *66:* 269–272 (1976).

383 Rosenthal, H.L.; Pfluke, M.L., and Buscaglia, S.: A stable iron reagent for determination of cholesterol. J. Lab. clin. Med. *50:* 318–322 (1957).

384 Ross, A.C. and Zilversmit, D.B.: Chylomicron remnant cholesteryl esters as the major constituent of very low density lipoproteins in plasma of cholesterol fed rabbits. J. Lipid Res. *18:* 169–181 (1977).

385 Rouser, G.; Kritchevsky, G., and Yamamoto, A.: Column chromatographic and associated procedures for separation and determination of phosphatides and glycolipids; in Marinetti, Lipid chromatographic analysis, vol. 1, pp. 99–162 (Dekker, New York 1967).

386 Rouser, G.; Simon, G., and Kritchevsky, G.: Species variations in phospholipid class distribution of organs. I. Kidney, liver and spleen. Lipids *4:* 599–605 (1969).

387 Rudel, L.L. and Morris, M.D.: Determination of cholesterol using o-phthalaldehyde. J. Lipid Res. *14:* 364–366 (1973).

388 Rudel, L.L.; Morris, M.D., and Felts, J.M.: The transport of exogenous cholesterol in the rabbit. I. Role of cholesterol ester of lymph chylomicra and lymph very low density lipoproteins in absorption. J. clin. Invest. *51:* 2686–2692 (1972).

389 Rudney, H.: The synthesis of β-hydroxy-β-methylglutaric acid in rat liver homogenates. J. Am. chem. Soc. *76:* 2595–2596 (1954).

390 Salen, G.; Ahrens, E.H., jr., and Grundy, S.M.: Metabolism of β-sitosterol in man. J. clin. Invest. *49:* 952–967 (1970).

391 Salkowski, E.: Kleinere Mitteilungen physiologisch-chemischen Inhalts (II). Pflügers Arch. ges. Physiol. *6:* 207–222 (1872).

392 Samuel, P. and Perl, W.: Long-term decay of serum cholesterol radioactivity: body cholesterol metabolism in normals and in patients with hyperlipoproteinemia and atherosclerosis. J. clin. Invest. *49:* 346–357 (1970).

393 Samuel, P. and Lieberman, S.: Simplified method for the long-term study of turnover and body masses of cholesterol by input-output analysis. Am. J. clin. Nutr. *27:* 1214–1220 (1974).

394 Samuel, P.; Crouse, J.R., and Ahrens, E.H., jr.: Validation of an outpatient method for measurement of cholesterol absorption in man. Clin. Res. *23:* 423A (1975).

395 Schaffer, C.B. and Critchfield, F.H.: The absorption and excretion of solid polyethylene glycols. J. Am. pharm. Ass. *36:* 152–157 (1947).

396 Schneider, H.; Morrod, R.S.; Colvin, J.S., and Tattrie, N.H.: The lipid core model of lipoproteins. Chem. Phys. Lipids *10:* 328–353 (1973).

397 Schoenheimer, R.: Methodik zur quantitativen Trennung von ungesättigten und gesättigten Sterinen. Hoppe-Seyler's Z. physiol. Chem. *192:* 77–86 (1930).

398 Schoenheimer, R. und Dam, H.: Über die Spaltbarkeit und Löslichkeit von Sterindigitoniden. Hopple-Seyler's Z. physiol. Chem. *215:* 59–63 (1933).

399 Schoenheimer, R. and Sperry, W.M.: A micromethod for the determination of free and combined cholesterol. J. biol. Chem. *106:* 745–760 (1934).

400 Schreibman, P.H. and Ahrens, E.H., Jr.: Sterol balance in hyperlipidemic patients after dietary exchange of carbohydrates for fat. J. Lipid Res. *17:* 97–106 (1976).

401 Schumaker, V.N. and Adams, G.H.: Circulating lipoproteins. Annu. Rev. Biochem. *38:* 113–136 (1969).

402 Scow, R.O.; Blanchette-Mackie, E.J., and Smith, L.C.: Role of capillary endothelium

in the clearance of chylomicrons. A model for lipid transport from blood by lateral diffusion in cell membranes. Circulation Res. *39:* 149–162 (1976).

403 Searcy, R.L. and Bergquist, L.M.: A new colour reaction for the quantitation of serum cholesterol. Clin. chim. Acta *5:* 192–199 (1960).

404 Shapiro, D.J. and Rodwell, V.W.: Diurnal variation and cholesterol regulation of hepatic HMG-CoA reductase activity. Biochim. biophys. Res. Commun. *37:* 867–872 (1969).

405 Shapiro, D.J.; Imblum, R.L., and Rodwell, V.W.: Thin layer chromatographic assay for HMG–CoA reductase and mevalonic acid. Analyt. Biochem. *31:* 383–390 (1969).

406 Shefer, S.; Hauser, S.; Lapar, V., and Mosbach, E.H.: HMG–CoA reductase of intestinal mucosa and liver of the rat. J. Lipid Res. *13:* 402–412 (1972).

407 Shefer, S.; Nicolau, G., and Mosbach, E.H.: Isotope derivative assay of microsoma cholesterol 7α-hydroxylase. J. Lipid Res. *16:* 92–96 (1975).

408 Sheltawy, M.J. and Losowsky, M.S.: Determination of faecal bile acids by an enzymic method. Clin. chim. Acta *64:* 127–132 (1975).

409 Shimada, K.; Bricknell, K.S., and Finegold, S.M.: Deconjugation of bile acids by intestinal bacteria: review of literature and additional studies. J. infect. Dis. *119:* 273–281 (1969).

410 Shioda, R.; Wood, P.D.S., and Kinsell, L.W.: Determination of individual con-jugated bile acids in human bile. J. Lipid Res. *10:* 546–554 (1969).

411 Siakotos, A.N. and Rouser, A.: Analytical separation of nonlipid water-soluble substances and gangliosides from other lipids by dextran gel chromatography. J. Am. Oil Chem. Soc. *42:* 913–919 (1965).

412 Simmonds, W.J.; Korman, M.G.; GO, V.L.W., and Hofmann, A.F.: Radio-immunoassay of conjugated cholyl bile acids in serum. Gastroenterology *65:* 705–711 (1973).

413 Simon, J.B. and Scheig, R.: Serum cholesterol esterification in liver disease. Impor-tance of lecithin-cholesterol acyltransferase. New Engl. J. Med. *286:* 841–846 (1970).

414 Sims, R.P.A. and Larose, J.A.G.: The use of iodine vapor as a general detecting agent in the thin layer chromatography of lipids. J. Am. Oil chem. Soc. *39:* 232 (1962).

415 Siperstein, M.D.: Regulation of cholesterol biosynthesis in normal and malignant tissues. Curr. Topics Cell Reg. *2:* 65–100 (1970).

416 Siperstein, M.D. and Fagan, V.M.: Feedback control of mevalonate synthesis by dietary cholesterol. J. biol. Chem. *241:* 602–609 (1970).

417 Siperstein, M.D.; Chaikoff, I.L., and Reinhardt, W.O.: ^{14}C-Cholesterol. V. Oblig-atory function of bile in intestinal absorption of cholesterol. J. biol. Chem. *198:* 111–114 (1952).

418 Siperstein, M.D.; Fagan, V.M., and Dietschy, J.M.: A gas-liquid chromatographic procedure for the measurement of mevalonic acid synthesis. J. biol. Chem. *241:* 597–601 (1966).

419 Siperstein, M.D.; Jayko, M.E.; Chaikoff, I.L., and Dauben, W.A.: Nature of the metabolic products of ^{14}C-cholesterol excreted in bile and feces. Proc. Soc. exp. Biol. Med. *81:* 720–724 (1952).

Clinical Methods in Study of Cholesterol Metabolism   158

420 Sjövall, J.: Bile acids in man under normal and pathological conditions. Clin. chim
    Acta *15:* 33–41 (1960).
421 Sjövall, J.: Separation and determination of bile acid; in Glick, Methods of bio-
    chemical analysis, vol. 12, pp. 97–141 (Interscience, New York 1964).
422 Skinner, S.M.; Clark, R.E.; Baker, N., and Shipley, R.A.: Complete solution of the
    three-compartment model in steady state after single injection of radioactive tracer.
    Am. J. Physiol. *196:* 238–244 (1959).
423 Skipski, V.P. and Barclay, M.: Thin layer chromatography of lipids; in Lowenstein,
    Methods in enzymology, vol. 14, pp. 530–598 (Academic Press, New York 1969).
424 Small, D.M.; Dowling, R.H., and Redinger, R.N.: The enterohepatic circulation of
    bile salts. Archs intern. Med. *130:* 552–573 (1972).
425 Smith. L.L.; Mathews, W.L.; Price, J.C.; Beckmann, R.C., and Reynolds, B.: Thin
    layer chromatographic examination of cholesterol autooxidation. J. Chromat. *27:*
    187–205 (1967).
426 Snog-Kjaer, A.; Prange, I., and Dam, H.: Conversion of cholesterol into coprosterol
    by bacteria *in vitro.* J. gen. Microbiol. *14:* 256–260 (1956).
427 Sodhi, H.S.: Disposition of dietary versus endogenous cholesterol: in Cowgill and
    Kinsell, The fate of dietary lipids. Proc. 1967 Duel Conf. on Lipids, pp. 75–87 (US
    Government Printing Office, Washington 1967).
428 Sodhi, H.S.: Relative rate of absorption into lymph of dietary and endogenous
    cholesterol from intestinal mucosa and their significance. Circulation *46:* suppl. II,
    p. 276 (1972).
429 Sodhi, H.S.: Cholesterol metabolism in man; in Kritchevsky, Hypolipidemic agents.
    Handbook of experimental pharmacology, vol. 41, pp. 29–107 (Springer, Berlin 1975).
430 Sodhi, H.S. and Kalant, N.: Hyperlipidemia in experimental nephrosis. III. Plasma
    lipoproteins. Metabolism *12:* 420–427 (1963).
431 Sodhi, H.S. and Kudchodkar, B.J.: Labeling plasma lipoproteins with radioactive
    cholesterol. J. Lab. clin. Med. *82:* 111–124 (1973).
432 Sodhi, H.S. and Kudchodkar, B.J.: Catabolism of cholesterol in hypercholestero-
    lemia and its relationship to plasma triglycerides. Clin. chim. Acta *46:* 161–171 (1973).
433 Sodhi, H.S. and Kudchodkar, B.J.: A new hypothesis correlating metabolism of
    plasma and tissue cholesterol with that of plasma lipoproteins. Lancet *i:* 513–519
    (1973).
434 Sodhi, H.S. and Kudchodkar, B.J.: A physiological method for labeling plasma lipo-
    proteins with radioactive cholesterol. Clin. chim. Acta *51:* 291–301 (1974).
435 Sodhi, H.S.; Kudchodkar, B.J.; Horlick, L., and Weder, C.H.: Effects of chloro-
    phenoxyisobutyrate on the synthesis and metabolism of cholesterol in man. Metab-
    olism *20:* 348–359 (1971).
436 Sodhi, H.S.; Horlick, L.; Nazir, D.J., and Kudchodkar, B.J.: A simple method for
    calculating absorption of dietary cholesterol in man. Proc. Soc. exp. Biol. Med. *137:*
    277–279 (1971).
437 Sodhi, H.S.; Orchard, R.C.; Agnish, N.D.; Varughese, P.V., and Kudchodkar, B.J.:
    Separate pools of endogenous and exogenous cholesterol in rat intestines. Athero-
    sclerosis *17:* 197–219 (1973).
438 Sodhi, H.S.; Kudchodkar, B.J.; Varughese, P., and Duncan, D.: Validation of the

ratio method for calculating absorption of dietary cholesterol in man. Proc. exp. Biol. Med. *145:* 197–211 (1974).

439 Sodhi, H.S.; Kudchodkar, B.J.; Salel, A.F., and Mason, D.T.: Differences in the hepatic metabolism between the endogenous and particulate cholesterol injected i. v. in alcoholic saline. 4th Int. Symp. Atherosclerosis, Tokyo 1976, p. 121.

440 Sodhi, H.S.; Kudchodkar, B.J.; Salel, A.F., and Mason, D.T.: Disposition of newly synthesized cholesterol in the liver of rat. 4th Int. Symp. Atherosclerosis, Tokyo 1976, p. 235.

441 Sperry, W.M.: The relationship between total and free cholesterol in human blood serum. J. biol. Chem. *114:* 125–133 (1955).

442 Sperry, W.M.: Quantitative isolation of sterols. J. Lipid Res. *4:* 221–225 (1963).

443 Sperry, W.M. and Webb, M.: A revision of the Schonheimer-Sperry method for cholesterol determination. J. biol. Chem. *187:* 97–106 (1950).

444 Sperry, W.M. and Brand, F.C.: The determination of total lipids in blood serum. J. biol. Chem. *213:* 69–76 (1955).

445 Stahl, E.: Thin layer chromatography; a laboratory handbook (Academic Press, New York 1969).

446 Stanley, M.M. and Cheng, S.H.: Excretion from the gut and gastrointestinal exchange studied by means of the inert indicator method. Am. J. dig. Dis. *2:* 628–642 (1957).

447 Steihl, A.; Czygan, P., and Raedsch, R.: Sulphation of lithocholate in patients during chenodeoxycholate treatment. A protective mechanism; in Matern, Hochenschmidt, Bach and Gerak Advances in bile acid research, pp. 347–350 (Verlag Stuttgart, New York 1975).

448 Stein, O. and Stein, Y.: The removal of cholesterol from Landschutz ascites cells by high density apolipoprotein. Biochim. biophys. Acta *326:* 232–244 (1973).

449 Stein, O. and Stein, Y.: Surface binding and interiorization of homologous and heterologous serum lipoproteins by rat aortic smooth muscle cells in culture. Biochim. biophys. Acta *398:* 377–384 (1975).

450 Stewart, G.N.: Pulmonary circulation time: quantity of blood in the lungs and output of the heart. Am. J. Physiol. *58:* 20–27 (1921).

451 Stoker, D.J.; Wynn, V., and Robertson, G.: Effect of posture on the plasma cholesterol level. Br. med. J. *i:* 336–338 (1966).

452 Stokke, K.T. and Norum, K.R.: Determination of lecithin: cholesterol acyltransferase in human blood plasma. Scand. J. clin. Lab. Invest. *27:* 21–27 (1971).

453 Stolyhwo, A. and Privett, O.S.: Studies on the analysis of lipid classes by gradient elution adsorption chromatography. J. chromat. Sci. *11:* 20–25 (1973).

454 Subbiah, M.T.R.: Stigmasterol as internal standard for simultaneous quantitation of biliary cholesterol and bile acids by gas-liquid chromatography. Clin. chim. Acta *48:* 19–21 (1973).

455 Subbiah, M.T.R.; Tyler, N.E.; Buscaglia, D.M., and Marai, L.: Estimation of bile acid excretion in man: comparison of isotopic turnover and fecal excretion methods. J. Lipid Res. *17:* 78–84 (1976).

456 Sugano, M. and Portman, O.W.: Fatty acid specificities and rates of cholesterol esterificaiton *in vivo* and *in vitro*. Archs Biochem. Biophys. *107:* 341–357 (1964).

457 Sugiyama, T.; Clinkenbeard, K.; Moss, J., and Lane, M.D.: Multiple cytosolic

forms of hepatic β-hydroxy-β-methylglutaryl CoA synthase: possible regulatory role in cholesterol synthesis. Biochem. biophys. Res. Commun. *48:* 255–261 (1972).

458 Suld, H.M.; Staple, E., and Gurin, S.: Mechanism of formation of bile acids from cholesterol: oxidation of 5β-cholestane-3α, 7α, 12α-triol and formation of propionic acid from the side chain by rat liver mitochondria. J. biol. Chem. *237:* 338–344 (1962).

459 Sundaram, G.S. and Sodhi, H.S.: Color detection of bile acids on thin-layer chromatography. J. Chromat. *61:* 370–372 (1971).

460 Sundaram, G.S.; Singh, H., and Sodhi, H.S.: Thin-layer chromatographic separation of chenodeoxycholic and deoxycholic acids. Clin. chim. Acta *34:* 425–429 (1971).

461 Swell, L.; Bryon, J.E., and Treadwell, C.R.: Cholesterol esterases, IV. Cholesterol esterase of rat intestinal mucosa. J. biol. Chem. *186:* 543–548 (1950).

462 Swell, L.; Trout, E.C., jr.; Hopper, J.R.; Field, H., jr., and Treadwell, C.R.: Mechanism of cholesterol absorption. I. Endogenous dilution and esterification of fed cholesterol-4-^{14}C. J. biol. Chem. *232:* 1–8 (1958).

463 Swell, L.; Boiler, T.A.; Field, H., jr., and Treadwell, C.R.: Absorption of dietary cholesterol esters. Am. J. Physiol. *180:* 129–132 (1955).

464 Swell, L.; Trout, E.C., jr.; Hopper, J.R; Field, H., jr., and Treadwell, C.R.: The mechanism of cholesterol absorption. Ann. N.Y. Acad. Sci. *72:* 813–825 (1959).

465 Swell, L.; Trout, E.C., jr.; Field, H., jr., and Treadwell, C.R.: Labelling of intestinal and lymph cholesterol after administration of tracer doses of cholesterol-4-^{14}C. Proc. Soc. exp. Biol. Med. *101:* 519–521 (1959).

466 Sylvén, C. and Borgström, B.: Absorption and lymphatic transport of cholesterol in the rat. J. Lipid Res. *9:* 596–601 (1968).

467 Sylvén, C. and Borgström, B.: Intestinal absorption and lymphatic transport of cholesterol in the rat. Influence of the fatty acid chain length of the carrier triglycerides. J. Lipid Res. *10:* 351–355 (1969).

468 Szalkowski, C.R. and Mader, W.J.: Colorimetric determination of deoxycholic acid in ox bile. Analyt. Chem. *24:* 1602–1604 (1952).

469 Tait, J.F.; Tait, S.A.; Little, B., and Laumas, K.: The disappearance of 7-H^3-d-aldosterone in the plasma of normal subjects. J. clin. Invest. *40:* 72–80 (1961).

470 Tan, M.H.; Wilmshurst, E.G.; Gleason, R.E., and Soeldner, J.S.: Effect of posture on serum lipids. New Engl. J. Med. *289:* 416–418 (1973).

471 Tarbutton, P.N. and Gunter, C.R.: Enzymatic determination of total cholesterol in serum. Clin. Chem. *20:* 724–725 (1974).

472 Tavormina, P.A. and Gibbs, M.H.: The metabolism of β, γ-dihydroxy-β-methyl valeric acid by liver homogenates. J. Am. chem. Soc. *78:* 6210 (1956).

473 Taylor, C.B. and Gould, R.G.: Effect of dietary cholesterol on rate of cholesterol synthesis in the intact animal measured by means of radioactive carbon. Circulation *2:* 467–468 (1950).

474 Thompson, J.N.; Erdody, P.; Brien, R., and Murray, T.K.: Fluorimetric determination of vitamin A in human blood and liver. Biochem. Med. *5:* 67–89 (1971).

475 Tint, G.S. and Salen, G.: Transformation of 5α-cholest-7-en-3β-ol to cholesterol and cholestanol in cerebrotendinous xanthomatosis. J. Lipid Res. *15:* 256–262 (1974).

476 Tonks, D.B.: The estimation of cholesterol in serum. A classification and critical review of methods. Clin. Biochem. *1:* 12–29 (1967).

477 Treadwell, C.R. and Vahouny, G.V.: Cholesterol Absorption; in Code, Handbook

of physiology, vol. 3, sect. 6, pp. 1407–1438 (Am. Physiological Society, Washington 1968).

478 Truswell, A.S. and Mitchell, W.D.: Separation of cholesterol from its companions, cholestanol and Δ7-cholestanol, by thin layer chromatography. J. Lipid Res. 6: 438–441 (1965).

479 Tschugaeff, L. und Gasteff, A.: Zur Kenntnis des Cholesterins I. Br. 42: 4631–4634 (1909).

480 Usui, T.: Thin layer chromatography of bile acids with special reference to separation of keto bile acids. J. Biochem., Tokyo 54: 283–286 (1973).

481 Vahouny, G.V.; Weersing, S., and Treadwell, C.R.: Function of specific bile acids in cholesterol esterase activity in vitro. Biochim. biophys. Acta 98: 607–616 (1965).

482 Vahouny, G.V. and Treadwell, C.R.: Absorption of cholesterol esters in the lymph fistula rat. Am. J. Physiol. 195: 516–520 (1958).

483 Berge-Henegouwen, G.P. Van; Allan, R.N.; Hofmann, A.F., and Yu Paulina, Y.S.: A facile hydrolysis-solvolysis procedure for conjugated bile acid sulfates. J. Lipid Res. 18: 118–122 (1977).

484 Cantfort, J. Van; Renson, J., and Gielen, J.: Rat liver cholesterol of 7α-hydroyxylase. I. Development of a new assay based on the enzymic exchange of tritium located on the 7α position of the substrate. Eur. J. Biochem. 55: 23–31 (1975).

485 Lier, J.E. Van and Smith, L.L.: Chromatography of some cholesterol autooxidation products on Sephadex LH-20. J. Chromat. 41: 37–42 (1969).

486 Varma, K.G.; Nowotny, A.H., and Soloff, L.A.: Characterization of antibody to human phosphatidylcholine: cholesterol acyltransferase. Biochim. biophys. Acta 486: 378–384 (1977).

487 Vlahcevic, Z.R.; Gregory, D.H., and Swell, L.: Validation of isotope dilution technique for determination of bile acid synthesis in man. Gastroenterology 67: 1299–1301 (1974).

488 Vlahcevic, Z.R.; Miller, J.R.; Farrar, J.T., and Swell, L.: Kinetics and pool size of primary bile acids in man. Gastroenterology 61: 85–90 (1971).

489 Wallentin, L. and Vikrot, O.: Evaluation of an in vitro assay of lecithin: cholesterol acyltransferase rate in plasma. Scand. J. clin. Lab. Invest. 35: 661–667 (1975).

490 Waterfield, R.L.: The effects of posture on the circulating blood volume. J. Physiol., Lond. 72: 110–120 (1931).

491 Watson, D.: A simple method for the determination of serum cholesterol. Clin. chim. Acta 5: 637–643 (1960).

492 Weber, A.M.; Chartrand, L.; Doyon, G.; Gordon, S., and Roy, C.C.: The quantitative determination of fecal bile acids in children by the enzymatic method. Clin. chim. Acta 39: 524–534 (1972).

493 Webster, D.: The chromatographic separation of ester and free cholesterol in blood. Clin. chim. Acta 8: 19–25 (1963).

494 Webster, D.: The direct estimation of esterified cholesterol with a number of commonly used cholesterol colour reagents. Clin. chim. Acta 8: 731–743 (1963).

495 Werbin, H.; Plotz, J.; Roy, G.V. Le, and Davis, E.M.: Cholesterol – a precursor of estrone in vivo. J. Am. chem. Soc. 79: 1012–1013 (1957).

496 Whereat, A.F. and Staple, E.: The preparation of serum lipoproteins labeled with radioactive cholesterol. Archs Biochem. Biophys. 90: 224–228 (1960).

497 Wilkinson, R.: Polyethylene glycol 4000 as a continuously administered non-absorbable faecal marker for metabolic balance studies in human subjects. Gut *12:* 654–660 (1971).

498 Williams, C.H.; David, D.J., and Iismma, O.: The determination of chromic oxide in faeces samples by atomic absorption spectrophotometry. J. Agric. Sci. Camb. *59:* 381–385 (1962).

499 Williams, J.H.; Kuchmak, M., and Witter, R.F.: Purity of cholesterol to be used as a primary standard. J. Lipid Res. *6:* 461–465 (1965).

500 Wilson, J.D.: The measurement of the exchangeable pools of cholesterol in the baboon. J. clin. Invest. *49:* 655–665 (1970).

501 Wilson, J.D. and Lindsey, C.A., jr.: Studies on the influence of dietary cholesterol on cholesterol metabolism in the isotopic steady state in man. J. clin. Invest. *44:* 1805–1814 (1965).

502 Wilson, J.D. and Reinke, R.T.: Transfer of locally synthesized cholesterol from intestinal wall to intestinal lymph. J. Lipid Res. *9:* 85–92 (1968).

503 Windaus, A.: Über die Entgiftung der Saponine durch Cholestereine. Ber. dt. Chem. Ges. *42:* 238–246 (1909).

504 Windaus, A.: Über den Gehalt normaler und atheromatoser Aorten an Cholesterine und Cholesterinestern. Hoppe-Seyler's Z. physiol. Chem. *67:* 174–176 (1910).

505 Windaus, A.: Die Konstitution des Cholesterins. Nach. Kgl. Ges. Wiss. Göttingen, Math-Physik Kl., pp. 237–254 (1919).

506 Windaus, A.: Über die Konstitution des Cholesterins und der Gallensäuren. Hoppe-Seyler's Z. physiol. Chem. *213:* 147–187 (1932).

507 Wollenweber, J.; Kottke, B.A., and Owen, C.A., jr.: Quantitative thin layer chromatography of chenodeoxycholic acid and deoxycholic in human duodenal contents. J. Chromat. *24:* 99–105 (1966).

508 Wollenweber, J.; Kottke, B.A., and Owen, C.A., jr.: Pool size and turnover of bile acids in six hypercholesterolemic patients with and without administration of nicotinic acid. J. Lab. clin. Med. *69:* 584–593 (1967).

509 Wood, P.D.S.: Absorption of labelled cholesterol: studies in human subjects; in Cowgill and Kinsell, The fate of dietary lipids, pp. 67–74 (US Government Printing Office, Washington 1967).

510 Wood, P.D.S. and Weizel, A.: Mass determination by direct weighing in estimation of cholesterol specific activity. Clin. chim. Acta *26:* 539–546 (1969).

511 Wright, L.A.; Tonks, D.B., and Allen, R.H.: Determination of cholesterol with special reference to the use of *p*-toluenesulfonic acid. Clin. Chem. *6:* 243–253 (1960).

512 Wuthier, R.E.: Purifications of lipids from non-lipid contaminants on Sephadex bead columns. J. Lipid Res. *7:* 558–561 (1966).

513 Wybenga, D.R.; Pileggi, V.J.; Dirstine, P.H., and Digiorgio, J.: Direct manual determination of serum total cholesterol with a single stable reagent. Clin. Chem. *16:* 990–984 (1970).

514 Yokoyama, A. and Zilversmit, D.B.: Particle size and composition of dog lymph chylomicrons. J. Lipid Res. *6:* 241–246 (1965).

515 Youmans, J.B.; Wells, H.S., and Donley, D.: The effect of posture (standing) on the serum protein concentration and colloid osmotic pressure of blood from the foot in relation to the formation of edema. J. clin. Invest. *13:* 447–459 (1934).

516 Zaffaroni, A.; Hechter, O., and Pincus, G.: Adrenal conversion of ^{14}C-labelled cholesterol and acetate to adrenal cortical hormones. J. Am. chem. Soc. *73:* 1390–1391 (1951).

517 Zak, B.: Cholesterol methodologies: a review. Clin. Chem. *23:* 1201–1214 (1977).

518 Zak, B.; Dickenman, R.C.; White, E.G.; Burnett, H., and Cherney, P.J.: Rapid estimation of free and total cholesterol. Am. J. clin. Path. *24:* 1307–1315 (1954).

519 Zak, B. and Epstein, E.A.: A study on several colour reactions for the determination of cholesterol. Clin. chim. Acta *6:* 72–78 (1961).

520 Zeitman, B.B.: Rapid method for determining free and esterified cholesterol in plasma extracts. J. Lipid Res. *6:* 578–580 (1965).

521 Zilversmit, D.B.: The design and analysis of isotope experiments. Am. J. Med. *29:* 832–848 (1960).

522 Zilversmit, D.B.: The surface coat of chylomicrons: lipid chemistry. J. Lipid Res. *9:* 180–192 (1968).

523 Zilversmit, D.B.: A single blood sample dual isotope method for the measurement of cholesterol absorption. Proc. Soc. exp. Biol. Med. *140:* 862–865 (1972).

524 Zilversmit, D.B. and Hughes, L.B.: Validation of a dual-isotope plasma ratio method for measurement of cholesterol absorption in rats. J. Lipid Res. *15:* 465–473 (1974).

525 Zilversmit, D.B.; Courtice, F.C., and Fraser, R.: Cholesterol transport in thoracic duct lymph of the rabbit. J. Atheroscler. Res. *7:* 319–329 (1967).

526 Zlatkis, A. and Zak, B.: Study of a new cholesterol reagent. Analyt. Biochem. *29:* 143–148 (1969).

527 Zlatkis, A.; Zak, B., and Boyle, A.J.: A new method for the direct determination of cholesterol. J. Lab. clin. Med. *41:* 486–492 (1953).

528 Zurkowski, P.: A rapid method for cholesterol determination with a single reagent. Clin. Chem. *10:* 451–453 (1964).

Subject Index